"This book provides a wonderful guide to elevating self-worth and getting aligned with your soul's purpose."

MELISSA AMBROSINI, AUTHOR, PODCASTER, SPEAKER

PS I LOVE *Me*

12 STEPS FOR A SELF-LOVE TRANSFORMATION

GINA SWIRE

PS I LOVE ME

First published in 2021 by

Panoma Press Ltd
48 St Vincent Drive, St Albans, Herts, AL1 5SJ, UK
info@panomapress.com
www.panomapress.com

Book layout by Neil Coe.

978-1-784529-58-1

Your intuition brought you here.

TESTIMONIALS

"This book provides a wonderful guide to elevating self-worth and getting aligned with your soul's purpose."

Melissa Ambrosini, author, podcaster, speaker

"Gina teaches you how to feel good in your own skin, set healthy boundaries and remove any obstacles to living a joy-filled life."

Jessica Huie, author of *Purpose*

"If you're looking for a way to genuinely love yourself without having the ick, you need Gina Swire. If you've wanted to really love yourself but don't know where to begin, this book is for you."

Sarah Powell, founder of Celebrate Yourself

"Gina offers us an honest and insightful exploration of what emotional health is all about, with powerful prompts to develop self-awareness providing the building blocks to a whole new relationship with ourselves."

Suzy Reading, psychologist and author of *Self-Care for Tough Times*

"Every woman needs Gina Swire in their life. Now, everyone can have instant access to all her wisdom in *PS I Love Me*. Gina has a unique ability to inspire women to love themselves and the steps in this book have played a crucial role in guiding me home to myself. Gina is the real deal!"

Kim Mellor, transformational coach

"This roadmap to self-love is packed with tools and techniques that can turbocharge a shift from the energy drain of low self-esteem to the revitalising energy of self-love."

Julia Shepley, women's coach

"Just like Gina herself, *PS I Love Me* wraps you in a cocoon of love and support. Each chapter is a clear step to falling in love with yourself."

Aimee Batuski, women's intimacy coach, retreat leader, and co-founder of Desire on Fire

"I love how effortless and fun Gina makes it feel to experience self-love. This book is a perfect gift for the women in your life."

Kelley Bode, women's intimacy coach

"Although Gina seemed to have the dream lifestyle when she was working as a plus-size model and travelling the world, she wasn't happy. This is a book about learning to love yourself – and we could all do with some of that! The 12-step guide is easy to follow and sensible, offering practical advice on learning to trust your intuition and manifest the life you want. Sounds good to us!"

Amanda Vlietstra, editor of *Chat It's Fate* magazine

ACKNOWLEDGEMENTS

I'm so grateful to my dad for all the sacrifices he made to support me and the continuous lessons I still get from him long after he walked this earth. He is my biggest teacher and the inspiration for my work. Even the name of this book was a gift from him, because his initials are PS. Call it a download from spirit.

I'm also profoundly grateful to my mum, who has supported me throughout everything, with whatever wacky ideas I've had and trusting my magic along the way!

I also want to thank the angels in my life:

Patricia Lohan, my mentor, who can give me one look and blast through a million limiting beliefs.

Miss Osha Key, who helped me extract all of my wisdom and make it into something with structure that others can absorb. Even in the hardest times, she is always there to offer humour and support.

Kris Emery, editor extraordinaire – thank you for your boundaries that taught me so much.

Juliet Catton, for instilling confidence in me and collaborating to add the final touches which reawakened my excitement in this book's long and winding journey.

My bestie Kim, for all the moral support and 'tech support' to bring this book to fruition.

Marta, my dear friend who I met in India, who then came to me in a meditation, years later, as the person to ask for support with the book. She originally read through my words and gave me so much encouragement. She was then inspired to write her own book, which she wrote and published before mine even came out!

And finally, I could not have made this entire book mission work without the loving care and thought of my amazing Self-Love Team. Thank you Donna, Mischa, Jen, Zoe, Juliet and Lily; you are angels in my life.

PREFACE

How this book got its name feels *very* important to me. And since the book is all about listening to these little voices and following them, it feels kind of cosmic to tell this tale.

I really wanted to include it in the book to show you that I practise what I preach, and that miracles are all around us!

Are you sitting comfortably? Then I'll begin… *hehe*. You can't beat starting a story with a good old 'dark night of the soul' can you?! I talk more about this later in the book.

I'd been in the deepest depths of despair. I was struggling to function at all, to be honest, and I'd not left my house for weeks. I had a pre-arranged meeting to go and pitch this very book to a publisher. I dragged myself to the train from Manchester to London and as I sat there, I begged my angels to help me. I felt horrific, like I was having a panic attack; my inner world was like an unknown territory and I couldn't think sharply like I normally would.

On the train I channelled something to say in the meeting and wrote it down in my notebook. I didn't read it through, I just trusted the download. When I arrived at the venue, it was a baking hot day, I was exhausted, sweating, and on the cusp of being late for this very important meeting.

I was annoyed because I didn't have a title that I loved yet, and I really wished I'd had the energy and capacity to work harder on my pitch. I loved myself through it, but it was still frustrating.

Then, *shock horror*, I suddenly realised that I'd left my journal on the train. Major FAIL. I panicked as I didn't remember anything I'd written down.

Just as I was walking into the meeting, I asked my angels to assist me. Instantly, I got the download: *PS I Love Me*!

I knew immediately it was the perfect name. There was no question, no 'let's sleep on it and see'. I knew that was *it*.

I went into the meeting feeling relatively sharp and when they asked if I had a title, I confidently said, "yes, I do, it's *PS I Love Me*." It felt so good and the reaction on their faces was a picture.

On the train on the way home I called my friend and said, "I got my title!!!!!" When I said the name, my friend said "OMG Gina, do you realise what this is?"

My dad is my main angel in the sky and his name was Peter Swire. PS! And in that moment, I knew more than ever that we are all being guided and that miracles are all around us!

Straight after that, I crashed out and had to sit out the rest of my dark night of the soul. But at least I had my title. And every time someone asked me what it was, their reaction was perfect.

It's my absolute honour to share this with you, as I welcome you to explore your own miracles through this book.

CONTENTS

➤–ᵛ–ᵛ–ᵛ–➤

And remember,
with self-love,

anything is possible!

INTRODUCTION

I want a large slice of that self-love pie!

"How did you end up being a self-love mentor?" It's a question I get asked a lot. But the question *behind* the question is this… How do you manage to love yourself fully and completely? How on earth do you *get there*?

In all honesty, I didn't always have self-love the way I do now. No, no, no. Don't be fooled by what you see now. And please don't compare your start to mine or to anybody else's middle! When I was younger, I went to a strict school that was very sporty and focused on academic results. It was all about playing first team netball or hockey and getting into Oxford or Cambridge. Running around AstroTurf chasing a ball with a stick was not my style and definitely not my path.

Even as a child, I wanted to talk about all things mystical, not boring linear stuff. And because of that, at some point, I started to believe that I had nothing important to say.

At school, I became very quiet, even though I wasn't a shy person at heart. Partly this was about negative self-talk. Most of the bad scenarios I played out in my head weren't real, but I was scared they would happen, so I hid. Then I went to sixth form, and life became all about partying. I came out of my shell a bit then, mostly fuelled by the booze culture. Going out, I became this super-confident person who was the life and soul of the party, who never wanted to go home, and who always wanted to be seen as having crazy fun. When I wasn't drinking, though, I would question everything. My looks, my intelligence, my confidence; I didn't think I had enough of any of it.

At 17, I was scouted for modelling, and part of me thought it would be great. But another part thought, *I don't think I can do this because if I'm the centre of attention, I won't be able to cover up my imperfections or my flaws.* I built up the courage to go into the agency in Manchester, and when I got there, they said, "We love you. You're absolutely great. We'd love to book you for a job. The only thing is, you're too heavy. If you go and lose a stone in weight and come back in two weeks, we'll sign you up."

This is common when you go into a modelling agency. And even though I'd been ill and lost a lot of weight, which was the reason I felt confident enough to go in there in the first place, they told me I needed to lose more. I didn't think I could do it. At the time, losing weight was the biggest thing in my life. I lived in a house where everyone was on a diet. Mum was always on a Weight Watchers or Slimming World diet, and when she was trying to lose a few pounds, I was doing it too. Me and all my friends were always trying to get skinny. It was just how things were. It was what I knew. But I didn't believe I could lose any more.

After the appointment with the modelling agency, I sat with my mum in Pizza Express having a salad, and she said, "If you really put your mind to it, you could lose the weight, but do you *want* to do it?" "I don't really want to be a model," I replied. "First, they ask me to go in, and now they're telling me I'm not good enough." So, that was that. I wasn't going to do it. But the Universe had a different plan. I was asked by two women who ran a smaller local agency, Karen and Sue, if I'd ever thought about doing any modelling. At first, I told them I was too big, but they needed curvy girls to model wedding dresses. "You'd be perfect for us! We want you curvy." And so, I started modelling after all.

One day, I was doing a job with a lovely makeup artist from the original agency that had turned me down. She sent my picture to the people she worked for, and the agency invited me back in to see them. "I'm not going back in there after they told me to lose weight!" I replied, but this time it was different. They wanted to take me on as a plus-size model. At first, I freaked out at that. "Oh God, I'm not going to be a fat model!" Then it got worse for my teenage self when the agency told me, "We love your face, we love your body, we love you. The only thing is you could be a bit bigger. Could you put on a stone in weight?" So, first they told me to lose a stone, and now they're telling me I need to put weight on. That was the last thing I wanted! What teenager wants to be bigger?! It was my worst nightmare.

Somehow, I signed up anyway and started doing jobs for this agency as a plus-size model. Sometimes, they put padding on me to make me bigger, sometimes they would choose the most unflattering shot, and sometimes the first time I would see a picture of myself was on the side of a bus or on a billboard looking bigger than I wanted. In my mind, I would think, *Oh my God, I'm so fat, I'm disgusting. I'm never going to be loved. I'm never going to find a guy who loves me because I'm bigger than everyone.*

Already you can probably see that a lot was going on at the time. I appeared confident, but underneath, I was really quite mean to myself. I was in a parallel universe. At home, I wanted to be skinny like my friends, who were all a UK size 6 –10. I created all these crazy habits, from going to the gym and eating only fruit to binge-eating. Then in my work life, I was the smallest of the plus-size models and was constantly being told that I wasn't big *enough*. It was so confusing.

Soon, I was signed in London and New York, and I started travelling all over the place. In the midst of feeling conflicted about my looks and my size, my career took off. As it did, my inner doubts continued. I always felt that modelling agency clients would only book me if no one else was available. I told myself stories that I wasn't beautiful enough, I wasn't curvy enough, I wasn't toned enough, I had too much cellulite. Yet nobody knew any of what was going on inside me.

As my career took off, I travelled more often and started living in New York. On the outside, it looked like everything was going brilliantly. But at the time, I wouldn't have agreed. I had amazing friends, was getting great jobs, travelling the world and being paid really well to wear gorgeous clothes and have my makeup done every day. I could buy whatever I wanted, and I partied like a crazy person! But I was deeply unfulfilled. The more unfulfilled I became, the more I would go out shopping and drinking, and on dates with men. I would alternate between eating really healthily and bingeing on anything and everything that I wouldn't normally allow myself.

I lived like this for years and never confided in anyone about how I truly felt. It seemed like I had it all. People would even message me on Instagram and say, "Oh my God, I want your life." And don't get me wrong. There *was* a part of me that saw how amazing my life was. I loved modelling and travelling, meeting people and experiencing so many different things. Yet I also felt fat, unhealthy and disconnected.

On a complete whim, I signed up for a nutrition course in New York. I wanted to learn about getting healthier, but instead I realised I'd bought a course on how to create a business to help *other people become healthier*. I'd messed up! Or so I believed… I decided to make the best of it and just do the modules that were interesting to me. Anything else, I wasn't going to bother with. I didn't have the time or capacity for anything extra back then. In all honesty, I was a bit burnt out. I had no time for anything except parties, modelling and sleep.

For the first few months of the course, I watched the videos about being healthy for yourself and realised health was not about food, which was where I'd been getting it wrong. Health was about knowing yourself, having awareness, loving yourself. As the course went on, I became more and more curious, and decided to do the other modules after all, following the breadcrumbs. Accidentally buying this course was the first glimpse that a little magic was happening.

At the same time, I didn't want to be modelling anymore. I kept having these thoughts about how modelling was all about creating an image that wasn't necessarily true. There's a big team around a model on a shoot. That team completely changes the way you look. On a shoot, you've got the best hair, the best makeup, lighting and photography experts, all working hard to create an image to make something sell. That's not how I look every day. Sometimes, the clothes I would model weren't even the clothes the company would sell. What if people were buying all this stuff thinking they were going to look like I did in the photos, but they wouldn't actually look like that because it wasn't even true?! It could make them feel like crap! It was not good for the planet. It was not good for humanity. And I just couldn't be a part of it anymore.

Yet, I didn't feel like I had any other skills. I'd been working my way up in this industry. I was at the top of my game. I had friends in corporate jobs who were climbing the ladder and earning good money, but I was just thinking, *Shit, if I leave modelling, what am I going to do?*

I was at a massive crossroads in my life, and partying harder than ever to distract me from it all. Finally, I took what was probably the biggest job of my career. I was on set in Manhattan when it struck me – everyone else wanted to be there, except me. It was like an out-of-body experience. You know those scenes in the movies? That was me. Standing still in the middle of the set, with everyone else buzzing around me. Something had shifted and I knew I couldn't continue on this path.

At the end of the shoot, I went straight over to tell my agent that I needed to go home to England. I just needed to get out of there. I was fully expecting her to say, "You can't do that," but she didn't. She was so good about it. She told me to take all the time I needed and to go and do my thing. Again, some magic was happening.

On the flight home to England that night, I planned to just chill out and watch videos on my laptop, but all my devices ran out of battery, every single one. So, instead, I took out a massive piece of paper from my bag, which I wouldn't normally carry but just happened to have, and mapped out what I wanted from my life. I remember asking myself questions like: *What do you really want? If money was no object, and time was no object, and you had all the support and connections in the world, what would you do with your life?* I divided my sheet of paper into sections and made loads of lists under different headings, like home, work, friends, travel, health. When I touched down in England eight hours later, I felt clearer than I had in years.

I also realised that I had never wanted to be a model in the first place. Sure, some part of me had, but it was more about the people around me saying I should go for it. As I look back now, modelling was a big part of my journey and I'm grateful for what it afforded me in my life, but there was something else at play…

Back in Manchester, I bought a house because having my own space was something I realised I wanted. I spent almost a year there just reading books, taking courses, doing yoga, learning to meditate and just being with myself. I didn't really go anywhere. I cut ties with a lot of friends. I went vegan and stopped drinking alcohol. And I deleted all the men from my phone that I used to just keep on the bench, just in case I needed some outside acknowledgement – the cheap junk food of love!

When I did this, the first thing that happened was I became incredibly isolated and lonely. The other thing that happened was my body dropped a whole load of weight within the first two weeks. It felt like shedding some kind of energetic protection from the men and the job that weren't serving me anymore. My body was closing the door on my career and old lifestyle. I had stepped away from it and now I really couldn't go back! I tried to leave the door open in case I needed the money, but now, as a UK size 12, I was the smallest I'd ever been, and returning wasn't even an option.

I was freaked out and unsure about what I was doing. But I was surrounded by the love of my family and, on some level, I knew it was what I needed. I had created this, and I had to guide myself forwards. I had no role model for what was essentially a spiritual path and personal growth journey. I was at rock bottom, on the floor and begging for a sign. Literally!

If you're reading this, you may recognise some of these ups and downs. And I want you to know something important. Rock bottom is truly a good place to be, because when you're at rock bottom, there's nowhere else to go but up.

And that's exactly what happened. As soon as I reached that point, I started to see interesting messages and I began to *trust*. These signs and voices became stronger and stronger. The first simple, yet powerful, message was this:

You don't need to change anything about yourself. You've been focusing on changing – on becoming more beautiful, more intelligent, earning more money. You don't need to do any of that. You just need to be who you are.

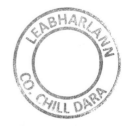

The next one was this:

**You are surrounded by love, but you've got no idea
how to receive it.
You've been loved your whole life, but you don't
have a way to accept it, so you feel like you need
more from the outside. You are looking for
acknowledgement, but when you are given it, you
push it away. In truth, you are so loved.**

The last big realisation was this:

**You want to be seen, heard, felt and acknowledged,
but love comes from within.
Your soul is free-flowing. You can tap into it at any
time. You are love and you are infinite.
You can give generously to everyone around you
and never run out.**

After a while on my own, I was a massive ball of love and people around me were starting to notice. They would ask, "What's going on with you? Whatever it is, I want a piece of that! Can you teach me how to do whatever you're doing?" I had no idea what they were talking about, but I did understand that a light had come back on inside me. I was radiating love and everyone around me was feeling it.

With my training in nutrition, from the course I had taken in New York, I decided that I would start coaching people around their health. It didn't take long for me to notice that none of it was truly effective if people didn't have a deep connection with themselves, AKA self-love. So, I switched to teaching people what I had learned from loving myself. But this turned out to be more of a challenge than I expected. I knew how *I* felt, but I didn't know how to teach it to other people. So, I packed my bags for a second time, and headed off to India to learn more.

In India, I found people who were very much on my wavelength. I'd made this shift and now I was attracting people into my life who were on the same frequency. I met so many amazingly free people who were travelling the world, loving themselves from within and sharing the message.

Finally, I felt like I'd cracked it! *This* was what I'd always wanted: community, freedom and love. It was weird experiencing all these feelings for the first time, while at the same time knowing I'd always had access to them. That's when I figured out how to teach people to love themselves; by becoming a role model. The role model I hadn't had when I'd been at my rock bottom. I knew this was my path. It had taken so long to figure it all out for myself but now I had all the tools and resources to help others. As well as an abundance of love to cocoon people in, whilst showing them just how good it could be.

And so… self-love mentoring was born!

In India, my mantra became:

I'm whole, I'm home, I don't need to change anything.

If anyone didn't like me the way I was, that was fine because it was just a reflection of them. I would only welcome people who got that. This was a revelation! I'd always been someone who needed to fit in and be liked, which had been so draining.

Only two short weeks after that, I fell in love with another person for the first time. It was incredible. I felt so good. I was doing something I loved, teaching people about self-love, whilst being in a relationship and travelling again. I took a flight to Bali and, before the plane had even touched down, I felt like I was home…

Fast forward five years, and after a whole lot of business mentoring, investing in myself, running an online business and practising self-love, I can tell you that this really works. I changed my life from being self-obsessed, seeking acknowledgement from the outside, constantly searching for *something*, pushing people away and never feeling fulfilled, to having a sense of self-love that comes with me wherever I go. I have distilled this learning into 12 essential steps to transform your life and walk the path towards truly loving who you are. I now hold self-love retreats around the world and live between the countries I love – all that outer freedom is a reflection of everything that has happened on the inside.

Everyone has bad days, and I still forget how great life is sometimes, but this is my story of remembering who I am and never looking back. These days, I love what I do. I feel like I have the secret to self-love; I've got the gift; I've uncovered the gold. And in this book, I want to share that endless abundance with you, too.

Why do we struggle to love ourselves?

Self-love is our natural state. It's the state into which we are born. It's when we're 'dropped in', when we get out of our head and into our body. It's when we're in high-vibe, natural and free. Self-love is the realisation that we are perfectly imperfect the whole time.

Often self-love does not feel like our natural state. Why is that? Sometimes, you'll hear people confusing self-love with narcissism. Narcissism is characterised by an inflated sense of self-importance, the need for excessive admiration or a lack of empathy for others. "She loves herself, that one," people say. Well, I'm here to tell you that the difference between self-love and narcissism is like the difference between self-worth and arrogance. They come from totally different places within.

Self-love is a completely different energy, even if it seems similar from the outside. In true self-love, you don't need external acknowledgement. Yes, it's nice to be seen and heard, but with self-love, you are overflowing with self-acceptance already, and that is the energy people receive. The energy of self-love is light and free, fresh and warm, loving and compassionate. It's about shining brightly and supporting those around you to do the same.

And here's the thing... Self-love is not about how it looks on the outside, or how *you* look on the outside, it's about how you feel on the inside. One day, I received a message on Instagram saying, "If I looked like you, I'd have self-love too." What this person didn't understand is that I looked like me 10 years ago, but I didn't feel the way I do now. How many attractive, successful, generous, loving, kind, healthy people do you know who can't see those traits in themselves? They just don't believe it. Everyone else can see their gifts, but they can't. Before I discovered self-love, I wasted what I had. I dimmed my light, like we're taught to do, and I missed out on the mystery and preciousness of life.

It makes sense that we've been taught not to stand out too much. Human beings evolved in tribal societies. There was an inherent risk of being cast out from the clan if a tribe member was perceived as different, which could have been life-threatening. In more recent history, wise women in command of their creative power risked being killed if they were outspoken. Ancestrally, our grandmothers, and the women who came before them, were right to tell us to dim our brightness; shining our light and owning our power could have been dangerous. However, in the world we live in today, I believe it is safe to shine. And it's time to shine our lights as brightly as possible to inspire other women to do the same.

Self-love is about how you feel inside; the relationship you cultivate with yourself. If that loving inner relationship is lacking, it doesn't matter how beautiful your Instagram pictures are, how slim or toned your body is or how amazing you look in makeup and clothes. None of that matters if you feel like shit inside. The energy you give out and the energy people receive comes from how you feel within.

Despite all the teaching I do around self-love, I still get asked: *Isn't this just about self-care?* But it's waaaaay deeper than that. In fact, self-love comes before self-care, and often the reason we're not taking proper care of ourselves is because we don't feel worthy of love. Crappy self-care comes from a place of fear and lack. If we think we're not skinny enough, beautiful enough or smart enough we may feel unloved or even unlovable. We may end up sabotaging ourselves because we don't feel we are worth loving. However, when we reconnect to self-love, it makes us naturally want to do good things for ourselves. People who love themselves don't want to treat themselves badly; they want their needs to be met. When we start loving ourselves, we remember to see our health as a gift. We notice how our finances, relationships and work life improve as a consequence of self-love.

Rarely do we hear a young child saying that they're 'fat', 'useless' or 'not good enough'. As children, we have self-love. It's only when we get a bit older (especially in our teenage years, although it's getting earlier) that the conditioning starts. The message we receive through school, friends, marketing and social media is that it's necessary for us to change, to be different, better, to consume whatever we're told to consume. We start believing what other people are telling us – that we are not enough.

If we believe what people tell us we are, instead of trusting what we know ourselves to be, a downward spiral begins. The belief that we're not good enough begins to take root and, because of the way the human mind works, we seek evidence to support this belief. This creates a lower-vibe state where we attract more of the negative things we falsely believe. We reach a point where even if a million people said, "Oh my God, you're so beautiful, you're so smart", we would believe the one person who said, "You're ugly and stupid." We have filtered out the real truth, and our new truth becomes this messed-up, destructive message.

Over time, we come to feel unloved or unlovable. Self-love means *undoing* all the unhelpful messaging. Self-love is knowing that there is always love around us and inside us. People want to love us, but we've been unable to *receive* love because we've become disconnected. Before this disconnection began we played, we smiled, we embodied self-love. The self-love journey is the journey back home to this natural state of love.

It starts with becoming aware of the filters we've put on reality. If we've been filtering out the people who say how wonderful we are and attaching ourselves to the people who say the opposite, we can learn to shift away from this. Self-love means validating yourself instead. Even if it doesn't feel natural, even if it means transforming your beliefs 100,000 times a day, you can choose to love yourself. It starts as a conscious choice and it becomes the most beneficial transformation you'll ever make.

Now, if you're ready to find out how to do that, here are the 12 steps to a self-love transformation that underpin the rest of this book.

The 12 steps to a self-love transformation

This path to self-love has been tried and tested. It's most successful when there is structure, so that you can take it step-by-step. I've broken down my transformational tips, tricks, hacks and mindsets into the following 12 steps.

1. Self-worth

2. Forgiveness and letting go

3. Trust and intuition

4. Blocks and triggers

5. Emotions and the inner void

6. Understanding self-talk

7. Comparison

8. Body acceptance

9. Making conscious choices

10. Growing through relationships

11. Emerging from the darkness

12. Power, passion and purpose

These are the 12 steps you'll follow throughout *PS I Love Me* as you move towards greater alignment and attracting what you truly desire into your life.

What to expect from *PS I Love Me*

The purpose of this book is to help you experience self-love by following these 12 steps towards a life of self-worth, acceptance, letting go and trusting your path. It will give you the tools you need to understand yourself better and live more consciously in alignment with the person you are on the inside. It will help you release patterns around unhelpful attachment to acknowledgement from the outside. It will help you get in touch with your passion and your power. In essence, it's about removing anything that is clouding your love for yourself and bringing you into greater alignment.

It will take work, work that is powerful. You may uncover a mindset that changes the trajectory of your life. You may stumble upon a transformational shift any time you pick up the book and flip through a few pages. *PS I Love Me* is packed with tools that cannot fail to leave you changed. The very fact that you're reading this means you're in the right place, showing up for yourself and doing the work it takes. Just by picking up this book and opening it, you have taken a step towards creating alignment within yourself. And I'm super proud that you're here.

Throughout this book, you will see words that might require a little explaining. Where I refer to the Universe, you may have another name for it, such as God, Goddess, Source or Future Self. I use these words interchangeably to mean a higher power. Aligning with your higher power is where everything comes together. It's what feels good. It's what feels right. You'll come to know this feeling in your body as a *Heaven yes! Fuck yes, yes, yes!* This is where I hope to take you in these pages.

Sometimes it's easier to understand alignment by explaining what it isn't. Feeling out of alignment is when you feel a bit *meh*, out of sorts or stuck in indecision. You know when you make a plan, but you don't really want to do it? That's because it's not in full alignment. Maybe a part of you wants it, like when I sorta, kinda wanted to do modelling. Or maybe you're doing something to please people at the expense of yourself. Or maybe you're making decisions that are actually destructive, like turning up at a friend's house when you're on a health kick and letting them twist your arm into drinking a bottle of wine together. If you recognise this feeling of being out of alignment, of constant inner conflict, then you're in the right place. It's exactly where I was when I kept saying yes to what wasn't fulfilling me and seeking acknowledgement in all the wrong places.

Here's how I'd love you to feel by the end of this journey: experiencing an epic YES on every level!

Maybe you can think of a time in the past when you felt like this. Scientific researchers call it the 'flow' state. When you're in 'flow', you are aligned with your highest self. You choose well. You make bold decisions. You take good risks. You feel ecstatic. You're 'dropped in' rooted, grounded and guided. Everything just flows. By following the 12 steps to a self-love transformation, you'll be able to access this feeling all the time.

Alignment means everything is perfectly imperfect. When you're there, it feels like a match made in heaven, complete guidance, being in the right place at the right time, knowing good things are coming. It's an abundance of opportunities, ideas, creativity, spaciousness, the right people and the right options all finding their way to you.

A little note on how to use this book...

Even though I can be a total good girl, I can also be a bit of a rebel when it comes to taking courses, reading books and playing by the rules, so I wanted to spell out that there are no rules when it comes to reading this book. The 12 steps are a thematic guide to self-love and not necessarily sequential, unless you want them to be. In essence, I invite you to read this book how *you* like!

If you're someone who likes a little structure, I recommend spending time reading through each chapter and letting it land for a day or two while you do the reflection or journalling in each 'PS Here's Your Self-Love Medicine' section. The chapters also have

'PS I Love Me Practices', which include exercises you can do when the time is right, like when something happens or when you see a pattern repeating that you'd like to change. If you can leave a day or two in between each chapter, you'll probably have extra ideas and realisations as you go about your day, or things will come up where you can use these practices. That's how you'll get the most out of the book.

Then again, maybe you're like me... I'll read a book as fast as I can, focus on all the bits that excite me the most, and do the interesting exercises there and then. Other exercises, I won't do at all. And some of them, I will go back and do at the end, maybe more than once! That's why I don't love it when authors tell me how to read their book and why I don't want to do that to you. They don't know my personality, where I'm at in my life, how I learn or that I like to do things differently. And I don't know that about you. So, use your intuition to read this book however you please!

Speaking of intuition and reading what resonates, this book is written with women in mind, but everyone is welcome. If you feel it resonates for you, feel free to read it, learn from it and extract the juice from it! Whoever you are, you are welcome here. I've read many books that were written for men and it gave me such a fun insight into another world!

You can also take all this with a pinch of fun! Having some humour about it will change the experience for you. As I like to say, it's all a big cosmic joke. Throughout this book, you may go deep, probably deeper than you've been before. I'll ask you to look at parts of yourself and your life that you may have been avoiding. Shining your cosmic light on the darkness is where transformation occurs, but it's not easy. If you can find the fun, lightness, humour and playfulness along the way, you'll lift your vibration to attract better things into your life.

Lastly, I need to mention that it may take some time to reach a state of believing that the world is good. In the meantime, I ask that you trust the process, trust this book and trust the path to transformation that I'm guiding you along. I have been teaching self-love for many years and have helped thousands of women all around the world, through retreats in Bali, Ibiza and England, through courses, coaching and events, one-to-one and in groups. This process is tried and tested. It is what has enabled the transformations I made for myself as well as the transformations I've had the pleasure to watch unfold for countless clients.

Nobody is exempt from bad days. We all have them. And yet, the time it takes to get back into harmony is shorter when you follow this process in full trust. If you struggle with this, don't worry, because trust is one of the first steps to self-love transformation that we'll cover. All you need to do for the moment is know that you are in the right place, at the right time, with the right teacher.

Self-love medicine

Now I'm going to ask you to take two small actions that will make a huge difference to what you're about to read in the 12 steps to self-love transformation in the coming chapters.

The first is to **choose an intention** for how you want to feel as you read this book. For a moment, close your eyes and drop into stillness. Get into a space of feeling totally supported that you are in the right place, that you are doing well and that you are aligning with your mission in life. Now open your eyes and write down your intention. You can come back to this at any time.

The second practice is to **find a picture of yourself from when you were a child**, your little self, around five years old, if possible. Carry that photo around with you as you do this work.

Doing this has been amazing for me. Whenever I take out my picture and look at it, I think of how cute this little girl was. Who knew that this tiny, innocent, pure, beautiful, wonderful little child version of me was going to go on such a magical journey and travel so far? And I'm not just talking about travelling to new places, but the expansion within the self, the lessons, realisations and love. This is a powerful tool if you're prone to being mean to yourself. Try it! Get that picture out and try being mean to that little girl. It doesn't feel right, does it? It feels completely wrong. And it reminds you to stop being mean to yourself as a grown woman.

With that, it's time to begin your incredible self-love transformation. I guarantee that when you stop focusing on lack, imperfection, negativity and rejection, you will find an expansive, creative, energetic, swirling yumminess where you know you can create anything you want in the world. This is where true passion and purpose are born. You will never look back. I promise you that.

You *can* love yourself through everything that comes your way. Self-love is a choice you make to love yourself in your lowest lows, your highest highs, and everything in between. This book is going to show you exactly how to do that, step-by-step.

And remember, with self-love, *anything* is possible.

Gina xxx

CHAPTER ONE:

Worthy with Nothing

"You've always had the power, my dear. You just had to learn it for yourself."

L. Frank Baum, *The Wizard of Oz*

You, my love, were born worthy. I was born worthy. We are all born worthy. Every child enters into this life worthy. Nobody ever said to a newborn baby, "Prove yourself first. Get a flashy job, a rich devoted husband, a badass luxury house with a wine fridge, fifty gold bars in your safe and space for a pony, *then* we'll see how worthy you are." No. We don't say that to anybody, but sadly we often do say a version of that to ourselves. This type of judgment-based expectation prevents us from falling madly in love with ourselves. Self-worth and self-love are absolutely interwoven, so this is where we must start.

Often, we attach our self-worth to external factors. We tune into dismal, disheartening and destructive self-talk. We decide we are unworthy of love.

It's all
welcome.

How do we lose our self-worth? Why do we start seeking outside of ourselves? And why do we let people shoehorn us into being someone we're not? You won't be surprised to hear that it starts in childhood. And if we manage to come away with any self-worth intact, our teenage years tend to destroy whatever remains.

The purpose of this first step is to rediscover your self-worth by connecting to the tiny baby self inside you. Finding the 'you' that you were before you lost your connection to your self-worth, the you who is still in there, completely worthy, ready and eager to get reacquainted!

The marker of self-worth

We are all born inherently worthy, but as we grow older, we begin to give our power away by attaching our worth to things that are changeable, like how much money we make, our relationships, our looks or our weight. Self-worth is nothing to do with anything that can change.

Let's start by exploring what self-worth looks like when you do have it. Self-worth comes down to three consistent behaviours:

- Showing up for yourself
- Making choices that serve your highest good
- Choosing to accept who you are

Let's break these down to really understand the concept of self-worth and how to achieve it.

Abandoning versus showing up

Showing up for yourself – constantly and consistently – means both being in the game and *staying* in the game. It means choosing

PS I LOVE *Me*

self-love 1,000 times a day and not abandoning yourself. Through the good times and the ugly times, you keep going.

I know how hard this can be when you face challenges, but remember that you always have a choice. If you want self-love and you are faced with a challenge, it's about stopping to ask yourself what you need to choose to be in that love frequency. And, difficult as it is in the moment, it's about being thankful for your challenges, because they are there to help you evolve. Focusing on gratitude can be a really self-loving act all on its own. This is a simple practice that you can choose anytime to improve your experience.

When shit hits the fan, most of us will abandon ourselves. We might think we've ruined everything and head to the fridge, or get absolutely plastered, or – if you're like I used to be – go online and shop, shop, shop to numb your feelings. Showing up for ourselves means being more conscious with our actions. When done consciously, there's nothing wrong with having a glass of wine if you feel stressed or shopping for a new outfit to feel good. It's not about judging that behaviour. It's about identifying when and how we abandon ourselves.

Here's an example. Imagine something really bad happens, and you face a huge challenge like losing your job. Abandoning yourself might look like negative thoughts: "I'm a worthless piece of shit. My boss was right to sack me. I'm rubbish and useless." Another way to think of this is if a friend did something wrong and really messed up, and your reaction was to abandon them, saying things like, "You're an idiot. Don't even speak to me. I don't want to see you. You should be ashamed of yourself!" In other words, abandoning yourself is like being a bad friend to yourself. A best friend would show up for you, wouldn't they? Their reaction to you messing up would probably be more compassionate, such as saying, "I can see what you've done. I can see why you've done it.

It sucks, but let's work it out together. Let me help you get through this, let me hold your hand, let me support you." What kind of friend do you want to be to yourself?

Making good choices

When you make good choices for yourself, you start to align with your highest good. If you make unhelpful, negative or ineffective choices for yourself, you align with your lowest potential. Nobody wants to be that person, because frankly that sucks, and we don't want that.

The great part about making better choices is that it's a *virtuous* cycle. As you start to make better choices, your self-worth increases because you choose yourself more and more. And as we have seen, choosing yourself *is* self-worth. Equally, when your self-worth increases, you will *want* to make better choices. And so, it continues.

PS I Love Me Practice

For one day, notice what happens as a result of making one good choice.

1. Choose a morning practice to set you up for the day, such as doing some Kundalini yoga, listening to a high-vibe podcast or meditation or having a dance party for one.

2. Wake up and do your practice of choice first thing. After you make that choice, you may notice that you feel good about yourself.

3. For the rest of the day, notice what other high-vibe choices you make and note them down.

> Examples: I had a choice about what to eat for breakfast, so I chose something that made me feel energised. I smiled more and was open to interactions throughout the day. I reached out to a friend and had a great conversation.
>
> When you made a good choice in the first instance, did you continue to make better, healthier choices that were aligned with how you want to feel within yourself and in your body, instead of choosing things that left you feeling tired and *meh*?

Choices are how you vote for your own vision. When I first became interested in veganism and eco-friendly living, I shared memes that said things like 'vote with your fork', because choosing what you eat is a way of voting for how you want the world to be. Making choices for your highest good is exactly the same. With each choice, you vote for yourself, your lifestyle, your vision of who you are, who you can be and who you will be. Your choices show that you care.

What do you need to choose or let go of to be in that self-loving frequency, AKA your natural state?

Choosing acceptance

The third sign of self-worth is the knowledge that you don't have to chase worthiness. You just have to tune in, because you are already so worthy. Simply knowing this may be enough to shift into self-worth and come home to who you truly are.

Acceptance is also about being okay with the fact that sometimes we all have shitty days, just as we all have phenomenal days. This ebb and flow are divine, and it is all serving us. Even when we do or say a stupid thing, forget the path we are on or lose our way for a while, it's okay. We are still worthy.

We can also tune into the worth of others as a quick way to reconnect with our own sense of self-worth. Even when our family, friends, partner or colleagues are flawed, we are still able to see that they are worthy. So, practise seeing the beauty, value and worthiness in other people to help you level up your own sense of worthiness. Because if you can align with the idea that loved ones are flawed but still worthy, you can align with the idea that you are flawed but still worthy.

One note on this: I'm not suggesting that you compare yourself to others by evaluating your mistakes in relation to other people's or compare what you have with what other people have. As you will see in Chapter 7, comparison is not the place to find joy, nor is it the place to find worthiness. The exercise above is about *seeing the beauty in other people* and knowing it is a reflection of what is within you. It is your beauty, your worth, being reflected back.

Worthiness comes from within

Do you attach your worth to external possessions or situations? Your bank balance? Your relationship status? Your home surroundings? Your career success? If the answer is yes, you need to know that your worth does not rely on anything outside of you. It comes down solely and exclusively to how you feel about yourself. You need to *feel* your worth, not own it or possess it.

If you need proof of this, think about the unhappy rich people you may have seen, the ones who *have it all* on the outside, but haven't figured it out on the inside. Please know that you can be rich, successful and happy, but the first step is not becoming rich in order to be happy; it's creating peace in your inner world and coming into alignment with your sense of worth.

When it comes to how to approach self-worth, the concept of needing to 'up' your self-worth is a trap. By 'trying' we've missed the point, which is to *tune in* to what's *already* here. Worthiness is self-sourcing, like a self-saucing pudding... yum! It's only when we start to source our worthiness from within, not from outside (which is always in flux) that we can truly understand our power, become magnetic and attract what we want.

Now that women are more empowered than ever before, and there are so many lady bosses (myself included), a new issue has arisen – and I have definitely fallen into this trap myself – judging ourselves through a traditionally masculine lens. Evaluating ourselves against what we have, how good we are at providing, how independent we are, how bold we are at driving our businesses forward. This leads us to forget or undervalue our other gifts, such as how nurturing, flowing and compassionate we are, our ability to multitask, nest, create a home, and the small fact that we have wombs, energetic or otherwise.

Forgetting to recognise these gifts began to affect my self-worth. Each human being has a polarity between two essential forces – an active 'go get it' energy and a softer, more receptive energy. I wanted to attract a partner who had a 'go get it' energy to match mine, but, because I was already giving off so much of this energy, I kept magnetising men who had longer, shinier hair than I did, and as much drive as a city centre apartment. I couldn't work out what on earth was going on! I'd started to believe that I wasn't hot enough, rich enough or powerful enough at business to attract the sexy catches, but after sitting with it I realised that wasn't it at all, thank Goddess! I just needed to take a chill pill and drop into my powerful, magnetic feminine essence. By reconnecting to the softer, more receptive parts of me, I was able to get back into alignment and magnetise a sexy, hunky, powerful partner who was also in alignment. As I'm writing this, I'm giggling, because my partner is currently downstairs preparing a slow-cooked bolognese while I receive this transmission straight from Source. I love it. We *can* have it all!

Even with nothing – even without my looks, my business, my family, my money, my quick wit – I am worthy of *true love*. I am the gift. My full range of attributes are a gift to the world. And so are yours.

Lacking self-worth

Where does it all start? That we think nobody likes us? That we experience self-doubt? That we lack direction? That we're scared of life? According to Doctor of Psychology Suzanne Lachmann, writing in *Psychology Today*, there are infinite places that we lose our self-esteem as we grow up. She summarises the sources of low self-esteem as:

- Disapproving authority figures (or belief systems), where you were criticised or told that nothing you did was good enough

- Absent or preoccupied caregivers who didn't pay attention, which can result in a belief that you aren't worth noticing

- Bullying coupled with unsupportive, over-supportive or uninvolved parents

- Academic challenges without support from caregivers

- Trauma, including but not limited to physical, sexual, or emotional abuse.

Lachmann adds that, while "the seeds of low self-esteem are sown elsewhere... society and the media make imperfections so immediately accessible, there is no relief from feelings of inadequacy", which compounds low self-esteem. This is the birthplace of seeking outside of ourselves, getting lost in comparison and feeling like we don't measure up. Yet, self-worth can *never* be sourced from anything that changes.

A number of years after quitting modelling, I decided to take it up again as a hobby. I didn't know why I was doing this, but I kept being asked to do modelling jobs in Bali, and because they kept coming across my path, I took it as a sign. I tuned in and asked, "Is this a yes or is this a no?" and I was surprised to feel that it was a yes, so I trusted the feeling and signed up with a modelling agency. I did one job and it turned out to be super creative, very unlike the kind of modelling I used to do. I could put my own spin on it, and I wore great clothes that made me feel good.

When the agency asked me to do another job and told me the rates, I realised how much my self-worth had transformed. I heard the low number and replied, "No, that rate doesn't work for me, so I'm not interested." Back at the height of my modelling career, I would never have done that, because my self-worth was so much lower, and I felt I needed to take every job because modelling was my career. When it became a hobby, knowing I didn't have to do it and that I had other income streams, I was able to advocate for myself more.

Here's what happened when I did. As soon as I'd said the fee didn't work for me, they replied with a number three times the original offer! I was on a call at the time so I didn't get a chance to reply to the message, but I thought to myself that it was cool that I would earn three times as much income just by standing up for myself. By the time I finished the call, I had another message from the agent, because I hadn't replied straight away. It said, "Okay, okay, I've spoken to them and we've sorted the fee." In the end, it was 10 times the original rate.

Going back to modelling showed me the growth I had gone through over that period of time and all the areas where I was no longer willing to give away my power.

Love comes from within.

Your soul is free-flowing.
You can tap into it at any time.
You are love, you are infinite.
You can give generously to
everyone around you
and never run out.

PS I Love Me
www.ginaswire.com

Now that you know what it looks like when self-worth is present in your life, let's look at how a lack of self-worth may show up in your life:

- Experiencing negative self-talk all day every day

- Experiencing self-doubt

- Thinking nobody likes you

- Believing everything other people say

- Lacking direction

- Feeling like you don't have what it takes

- Thinking people are deliberately trying to hurt you

- Comparing yourself to others

- Feeling unacknowledged by others

- Wishing your body was different

- Wishing you had a different life

- Feeling like a spectator rather than a player in the game

- Not feeling chosen

Some of these may be difficult to admit or even notice. You may not catch yourself actually thinking, *nobody likes me*, but it might still play out in behaviours such as people-pleasing and letting people walk all over you. Here are some tell-tale signs that you're lacking self-worth and it's having an impact on your life:

- Allowing others to push you in a certain direction

- Being scared to ask for a pay rise

- Having shitty boundaries

- Letting people take advantage of your time or money
- Charging low rates
- Doing what is easy rather than what is fulfilling
- Scrolling excessively
- Being too shy to approach someone to talk to
- Waiting for men to pick you or choose you

You'll notice that a lot of these come down to not having the courage to speak up for yourself and what you stand for, or needing validation in order to do something.

Validation

Realising that I didn't need validation or permission from others caused a massive shift away from the above ways of thinking, into a space where I value and validate myself. It's cringey to think about it now, but I used to give away my power all the time: posting pictures on social media and waiting to see if people thought I was beautiful, outsourcing my power to men or to modelling clients.

When you love yourself, you're not dependent on others for love, but you still want to be seen, heard and appreciated. That is natural in humans. However, wanting to be seen, heard and appreciated is very different from desperation. With self-worth, your life doesn't depend on other people's approval. Attention is not your intention. Paradoxically, when you are not attached to the attention, you tend to get more of it.

PS I Love Me Practice

The 'cuteness' hack is a highly transformative state of mind that silences the inner critic, the attention-seeker and the outward validator.

Imagine you're on Instagram and you post a picture where you think you look good, hoping to get plenty of approving comments. Maybe you get some. Maybe you don't. Either way, eventually, the 'likes' dry up and self-doubt creeps in. You enter a downward spiral. You start thinking you're not good enough, and so on. Here's what to do when you notice yourself spiralling.

1. Take a step back and notice this is happening.

2. Realise your human self is simply trapped in her humanness. How cute of her!

3. Say out loud, "That's so cute. My human self just went into a little downward spiral of thinking she was worthless. It's all because her beliefs are trying to keep her small and safe. Isn't my human self so cute, experiencing all this stuff that she thinks is so scary?"

Your critic cannot exist when there is cuteness. Your little human self just needs a hug. That's why she's seeking validation elsewhere. Take out that yummy grandmotherly self-validating love for yourself and have some fun supporting your little human self.

If everyone was empowered...

If everyone was empowered, nobody would be going around trying to prove themselves by having more, more, more… Bigger, better, keeping up with the Joneses. The true power within us doesn't need to scream how powerful it is. It just quietly knows and doesn't need to prove anything to anyone. If everyone owned their power, the world would be a completely different place. Just for a second, let that truth land or take out your journal and fantasise about how the world would be different. That's a world I'd love to experience. I get to experience pockets of it in the conscious communities I live in. And I'd love for you to experience a world like that too.

I want to help a billion women overcome their inner struggles and reconnect with the innate self-worth available to all of us. I have taken up this mission because I believe that self-worth is our birth right and that the world would be a different place if we were all vibrating on this higher frequency, all living with passion and purpose, all overcoming the challenges that keep us negative and stuck. Self-worth gives each of us the space to create a ripple effect, and, when a billion people feel amazing from within, the whole world changes.

Consumerism, over-buying, over-eating, world hunger, animal cruelty, ocean pollution, not giving a fuck about things we really should give a fuck about, all this could be solved with self-worth. When we feel good, loving and worthy, we need so much less. We eat less, we buy less, we shop less, we desire less, we require less. And we simplify more.

If everyone was empowered, I believe the world would be a better place. Look at the impact of a simple self-worth choice. If one empowered woman does not get triggered by a situation over a man, she doesn't binge-eat a load of crap, which means she doesn't also consume the plastic packaging, which means that plastic doesn't end up in the ocean. If one empowered woman does not get triggered, she goes home and makes a nutritious joyful meal, connecting with other people, and the self-worth expands outwards.

Doesn't it feel good to zoom out and see why we're really on this self-love journey? You can always come back to this bigger picture if you are struggling or entering a downward spiral. When life gets a bit crazy, realising why self-worth matters can be so wholesome. Everyone stepping into their greatness and connecting to their genius would eliminate misery among people. It would harmonise and heal. Solutions to the world's worst problems already exist. We just need to feel worthy enough to use them.

The arrogance argument

If self-worth has so much power to harmonise and heal the world, why-oh-why-oh-why aren't we using it to our advantage? I am convinced that it's because we have long been confusing self-worth with arrogance.

People often ooze a fake sense of self-confidence because of how self-conscious they truly feel. This used to be me. Essentially, arrogance is self-consciousness dressed up in a really out-there party costume. True confidence doesn't need to prove itself.

Let's take a look at a few more definitions. According to the Cambridge English Dictionary, *arrogant* (adj.) means 'unpleasantly proud and behaving as if you are more important than, or know more than, other people'.

Unpleasant

The keyword here is 'unpleasant'. Like a flavour, taste or style, it is subjective. Unpleasantness is in the eye of the beholder. And so, a person can be arrogant, or they can be inspiring, depending on the perception of the beholder.

In my view, arrogance comes from a different place to self-worth. Arrogance has the angle of there not being enough to go around. It's like saying, "I'm so great and you're not" or, "I want people to know that I'm so great", whereas self-worth comes from a deep place of knowing our greatness, being humble and being prepared to use our gifts for good.

There is a fine line between self-worth and arrogance. Sometimes, people see others' self-worth as arrogance because they are not ready to see worthiness in themselves. It is a reflection of their own inability to make choices for their highest good and of the void within themselves that they can't conceive of self-worth being inspiring or for the greater good of all.

I'm not proud of this example, but I have been there myself. When I was growing up, I had people around me who would talk about others behind their back. If a woman walked past who was out of shape, wearing something ill-fitting or had crazy hair, I picked up on other people's back-biting behaviour and would add a similar comment. When I shifted how I felt about *myself*, I stopped judging others and began celebrating the joy of people showing up with confident, high-vibe energy flowing through them.

Now when I see people who are exuding a 'who-gives-a-fuck' vibe on the outfit front, it's inspiring for me. Unpleasant is in the eye of the beholder. In the past, I would have perceived someone's 'bad outfit' or 'crazy hair' as unpleasant, but fast forward to today and now I'd say, "Get it, girl!"

Important

Let's look at the other aspect of that definition of arrogance: thinking we know more than someone else.

We are all experts in different areas, depending on what we have chosen to dedicate our lives to understanding for ourselves, for our clients and for the world. When we want to master something, we try to imbibe all the knowledge and education we can, studying it like crazy every day and practising what we preach. We take a subject that we're passionate about and we learn everything there is to know. Simply knowing more than others about a subject isn't inherently bad, if it is demonstrated from a place of love. Indeed, that's how leaders and experts are born. Arrogance is a completely different intention.

Ultimately, it comes down to passion and inspiration. Personally, I want to hear about it if you're really good at something, because that inspires me. If you're great in bed, if you make a cracking lasagne or if you can do the best cartwheel anyone's ever seen, then please tell me that! I promise I'll never think, 'Who does she think she is?' I might have done in the past, but when a woman is empowered, she sees others' gifts as a blessing. Sharing those gifts and following our passion and our purpose is how we change the world.

Know this in your mind and feel this in your body... You are so inspiring, you are so amazing, you are so worthy, and you are so loved. You are completely cosmic. And nothing external can ever affect your worth.

PS Here's Your Self-Love Medicine

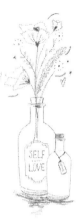

How would you want to be valued by somebody else and seen through their eyes?

It's your job to see yourself that way.

If everything you read in this book were to ramp up your self-worth by x 100, what would be different in your human experience? What actions would a super self-worthy person take if they were living your life?

If you are a perfectionist and don't wanna ruin the pages of this gorgeous book with your scribbles, I know, I've got you(!!!), head over to my website for some sassy AF printables that you can fill in and keep :-) along with some extra juicy self-love goodies, at www.ginaswire.com/bookresources.

CHAPTER TWO

A Clean Slate

"Sometimes the bravest and
most important thing you can do
is just show up."

Brené Brown

Before stepping fully into self-love, it's important to clear space for the goodness to come. Starting with a clean slate means learning to forgive and let go of the past, because holding on to old stories and blame means we are full of pain, which takes up space in our lives.

There are many powerful ways in which forgiveness can serve us. Not only does it help us create space for new visions and ideas to come into our lives, but it helps us understand how the past has served us, throws new light on our own perspectives, and even frees other people. Practising self-love through forgiveness makes the recovery from challenges shorter and helps you become stronger and more resilient as you move through life, so I urge you to be open to forgiving the hurts of the past, no matter how hard this might seem.

I'm whole.
I'm home.
I don't need to change
anything!

Forgiveness is incredibly powerful for setting us and others free. Even the *intention* to forgive somebody, even the *idea* of forgiving someone at some point in the *future*, has the power to create shifts. If you don't feel you can forgive a person for something right now, know that it doesn't have to be immediate or rigid. You don't have to know how or when you will be able to forgive someone. It's different for every single situation. And sometimes it's a case of forgiving the person or their wounded soul, rather than the action itself.

For now, as you move through step two of your self-love transformation, just trust the power and freedom in forgiveness and letting go.

All about perspective

When I was a child, something happened that really hurt. I went through my family breaking up and my dad leaving and starting a second family. As a young child, with a new half-sister and brother, I felt pushed out and abandoned. The way the breakup happened impacted my mum, which in turn had an impact on me. For all this, even as an adult, I hadn't forgiven my stepmum, who I felt was part of the reason it had all happened. In fact, I held onto the belief that one day she would apologise for everything she'd done.

A few years ago, I started doing this forgiveness work and realised that expecting an apology was ingrained in my own beliefs. Since I'd never do what she did, I thought she was wrong for doing it. However, I came to understand that the reason I would never do what she did was purely because that was what wounded me as a child. In other words, I would never do that because I have been the victim of it. On the other hand, my stepmum has had a totally different upbringing, totally different life, and dealt with totally different battles. What she did wasn't right or wrong. It was my perspective that was making it into something I felt she should apologise for, which was actually a way of holding on to pain and resentment in my own body, rather than letting it go and returning to harmony and love.

It was not really an apology that I was waiting for after all. Something inside me had to shift. I needed to forgive. So, I stayed up all night and wrote this huge, long letter, pages and pages and pages long. And here's the thing. The letter was not to give to her. The letter was addressed to her, but its purpose was for me. It was powerful in creating a shift. I stayed up all night, because I just wanted to get this out of me. The resentment had been in there, suppressed, for all this time, and it needed to be released.

Through the letter writing, I also realised a lot of the pain and heartbreak I felt around that time wasn't even mine. It was my mum's that I had taken on as a child without even knowing it. Now I'm an adult and able to understand this on an intellectual level, I have released this pain by exploring the feelings, forgiving and letting go. And that felt soooooooooo good!

Writing the letter would have been enough to let go and forgive, but here's the magical part. The very next day, having not spoken to each other for years, I received a text message from my stepmum. How about that for a big cosmic joke? There was no explanation for her getting in touch, but I knew it was because I was doing the inner work.

Holding on to all that anger, sadness, hurt, expectation and need for her to validate my experience wasn't helping me (or anyone). It was hindering me, weighing me down and holding me back. It was giving me the feeling of having to wait for something in this situation, which was then mirrored out into my whole life too. I was giving my power away to her, but we can empower ourselves by letting go and transmuting past hurt into love. Forgiving my stepmum, and myself for the role I played, was therefore a huge act of self-love.

Imagine for a second that we are all connected by invisible cords. When I pull on a cord, somebody else feels it. Have you ever been newly single when, out of the blue, a prior ex gets in contact? They know! It happened to me once when three men from my past all 'checked in' with me the same day I broke up with someone, without me saying anything or posting on social media. It's crazy in a way, but logical when we study energy. What affects one person affects all humans.

After I forgave my stepmum, I also forgave myself. After all, I was the one who'd been holding on to this for all these years: creating issues in my own life and sending out negative energy. It was all for good reason though. Maybe I would never have become a self-love fanatic or written this book if these lessons hadn't come my way! That's why I'm grateful for everything that happens. As my mum says, "Oh Gina, it's all character-building." I used to respond to her, "Mum, for God's sake, my character is built!" Little did I know, I had many more bricks to lay.

The space for new good things

"Resentment is like taking poison and waiting
for the other person to die."
Malachy McCourt

Often, when we think about forgiveness, we think of forgiving others, but sometimes it's about forgiving ourselves for allowing other people to treat us the way they did. The practice of forgiveness is for you, because holding on to pain, anger or resentment towards someone else is causing *you* harm, not them. Forgiveness of yourself and others is a gift you give yourself, because it frees you from the pain you've been harbouring.

When we forgive ourselves, or someone else, for something we perceive as having *happened to us*, we clear space for amazingly good things to come into our lives, which is why forgiveness is a fantastic foundational practice for self-love. In every workshop, retreat and training that I run, forgiveness comes up, because it is so fundamental. Even if you did just this one step, you would invite massive expansion into your life and self-love (though I'm not saying only do this one step! Please do all 12 for maximum expansion!). When we clear out old resentments that are keeping us stuck, we create space for new visions to come in, for ideas to flow and for deep, infinite, juicy, divine love to enter. Yey!

The energetic bonus of reciprocity

Often, a powerful, magical side effect of setting yourself free from resentment is that you tend to set the other person free as well. You create spaciousness in your own life, but as a fun little energetic bonus, you release the other person too. This act of self-love in setting yourself free has a ripple effect of love that extends beyond yourself (a lovely reminder that self-love isn't selfish!).

This exact synchronicity happened to one of my clients while we were on a retreat. This amazing lady was going into a new relationship and felt a little unavailable to her new partner. When we looked into why she was feeling this way, she figured out that it had to do with an ex-boyfriend and their relationship ending badly five years ago. A lot of horrible stuff had happened, and she hadn't forgiven him or herself. She didn't realise that she needed to forgive herself, because she was holding him responsible for all the blame.

When we did a lot of work around this over the course of a few sessions, my client made a breakthrough and realised that this resentment had been hurting her way more than it was hurting him. Forgiving him didn't mean 'letting him off the hook' either. When she had this huge realisation, tears rolled down her cheeks, a sure sign that she was releasing something.

The next morning, even though they hadn't spoken in five years, she received a text message from her ex saying, "Maybe we should have a little talk. I feel like I'm only just realizing how amazing you were and how wrong I was to you." Needless to say, she was in complete shock that this could happen.

In truth, this reciprocity makes complete sense. Let's return to the idea of everyone on the planet having invisible cords that attach us to each other. We are all interconnected. We are all one. When one person shifts their awareness or turns up the love frequency or levels up in some way, everybody feels it, which is good for mass consciousness awakening.

Moving resentment out of your body

When we're constantly dwelling on a story about something that happened – for example, my client with her ex-partner, how he wronged her and how she blamed him – it is incredibly draining on our energy. We know this. We know something needs to shift to free up space, but how do we even start? Forgiveness may be fundamental to self-love, but that doesn't make it easy, which is why I suggest starting with creating the conditions for forgiveness and locating where the resentment resides within you.

PS I Love Me Practice

Creating the conditions for forgiveness means coming out of the mind and dropping into the body. This embodiment practice is fantastic for exploring the way you feel about your past.

1. Start by getting comfortable and quiet. Bring to mind the person you feel anger towards or the issue causing you pain.

2. Then ask yourself:

   How does it feel in my body? Where does it hurt?

   See what comes to you. Nothing gets solved in the mind so try doing this without thinking too much. You might notice a lump in the throat. It might be tightness in the jaw. It might be a sensation somewhere else in the body.

3. Now, you're going to move this pain out of your body from wherever this resentment is stuck. You can move stuck energy out of the body by walking in nature, dancing or moving. I love to do it by shaking and growling, so if that calls to you, go and do that with the intention to release!

4. If you had trouble locating where resentment resides in the body, another way to move through pain is to use this journal prompt:

   I am yet to forgive myself for...

Put pen to paper and see what wants to be written. It could be something simple and small or it could be something major.

Whatever it is for you, make this a daily practice alongside gratitude, because doing this regularly can be a powerful way to release stuck energy.

Examples: I'm yet to forgive myself for not going to see my grandparents. I'm yet to forgive myself for lying to my friend. I'm yet to forgive myself for causing a huge drama.

Perceptions of the past

Forgiveness can be tricky, even when we start practising regularly, so I'd like to share another perspective that you might find helpful. What is the alternative to holding on to this blame, sadness, anger or disappointment? If you think about it, acceptance and letting go are the only truly self-loving options.

Blame and disappointment, or getting lost in sadness and anger, can create destructive, low-frequency states which impact all other areas of your life. If you're consumed with blame and resentment, how will you show up in a room? If you choose to let go, forgive and heal that part of you, how might you show up in a room then? If you choose to hold on to anger, how will you behave in your life? If you choose to let go, forgive and heal that part of you, how will you behave instead? Probably very differently energetically, right? When you hold on to these feelings, you hurt yourself more. And while the other person may feel something through the invisible cords between you, they probably won't be experiencing it like you are.

It's a story repeating. The trick to acceptance is reminding yourself that this repeating story *can* be changed, even though what happened in the past cannot. Present-day issues, challenges, problems or dramas that are related to a past grudge aren't going to change until you can change the way you look at it, the way

Self-love

is not about how it looks on
the outside, or how you look
on the outside, it's about how
you *feel* on the inside.

you feel about it, the way you relate to it. All that is in your power. Having this choice is the empowering part. And when you choose acceptance, you are practising self-love on the deepest level. You are saying, "This is what happened and I'm okay with that because I still like myself as I am."

Choosing acceptance

"As I forgive myself, it becomes easier to forgive others."
Louise Hay

Once you've done all this forgiveness work, how do you know if it has worked? How do you know when you've forgiven somebody and that you've grown the love you have for yourself in the process? The way I can tell I have truly forgiven someone is when I can think about that person or see them and feel neutral. I don't feel any of the lower-frequency emotions, like disappointment, fear, rage, misery, dread or blame. I don't feel like, "Oh my God, I'm still in love with that person." Or "Oh my God, I need to hang onto something from them." A middle ground exists of being okay with everything and knowing it was for my own good.

In other words, it's a different vibration, a more loving and compassionate vibration towards them *and* towards myself. When people say they need to get over their ex, let go of a belief system, or stop hating a part of their body, what that usually means is they need to accept and allow what the Universe is presenting to them. I used to think like this myself. I would say I needed to get over my ex. Instead of that, a much more powerful way to think about it is you might never get over that person. Do you even want to get over them? You know you have forgiven them when you start accepting the journey you are on. You may start asking a different question. How can I accept that this is just where I am?

By accepting and allowing, you will have a different kind of relationship with the problem or challenge. You release the resistance towards it. When you think, "I must let go", you focus on the need to let go. And when you focus on something, you only strengthen its grip on you. You manifest or attract it. That's not how to achieve letting go! True letting go is accepting; allowing whatever is there to just be there.

Acceptance is another aspect of empowering yourself. The best news is that when we have more compassion and love for ourselves and others, we need to forgive less often, because we stop judging people by our own standards and we can see that everybody is doing their best. The acceptance starts to happen at the time rather than attaching negative meaning and needing a forgiveness ritual.

One of my clients had been in a relationship that she knew was bad from the start. She realised early on that something was off, and the man turned out to be a narcissist who was playing games with her. He even said so! But she trusted the situation and let herself be sucked in.

A few years after this had happened, she was in a new partnership, but had still not healed her old resentments, so it had reared its ugly head and was causing havoc with her new guy. She worked with me for a while and kept talking about how she had to forgive the ex for what he had done. One day, realising she was fixating on having to forgive her ex, I said, "Have you forgiven yourself?" She had never even thought of forgiving herself and started beating herself up for being an idiot getting involved with him. She had a lot of resentment towards herself and her own choices, like, "I knew it was wrong. I knew what was going to happen. I shouldn't have gone there." All these heavy beliefs came tumbling out.

I'm telling you this because you can forgive yourself for all of that stuff too; accepting that you did what you thought was right or felt compelled to do in the moment. Sure, looking back, you may think that something you did in the past was really stupid, but you were doing your best with what you knew at the time. We can let go of the silly little things that we funny little humans do when we're in the moment, when we want love, when we didn't know better. Sometimes we get ourselves into situations that don't support our greatest good, but every wrong step is teaching us a lesson…

Challenges in the past have served you

Your past is a teacher, and you took a great lesson from it. It's all research for the life you want to live. It's a gift leading you closer to what you want. Maybe it's as simple as you just don't do that again. The idea that you have to 'get over it' or that it's 'not a big deal' is actually quite unhelpful when you look at it. You wouldn't tell someone to 'get over' a life lesson, would you? You wouldn't tell your best friend to stop whining and just get over something. Well, you might, but it would be good to be a bit more supportive. And this is exactly what we need to be for ourselves when it comes to 'getting over' some kind of trouble from our past.

Not only does it cause friction, confusion and upset when we're told to 'just get over' something, but we overlook the love and the good we once had. Take relationships, for example. Better to accept that the love we once had has shifted and may never be the same again, than 'get over it' and wipe it out. It is still love. It is still there. Love doesn't disappear, but love can change or take a different path.

Once you see this, you're ready for what comes next. If you are here reading this book, no doubt you have experienced some drama, some upset, some abandonment, some trauma in your life at some point. I want you to know that you are a brave soul, who has only faced challenges because you are ready for the next level. The Universe only sends us the challenges that we are ready to face. It may even be comforting to remind yourself of this when you are facing a challenge, because it shows you are ready for the next level of soul evolution.

Every time you are challenged, it's a lesson. Every time you face a problem, it's good for your evolution. Every time you create hardship for yourself, your soul is transforming, and you must be ready for it. The challenges you are sent equal the growth you must go through. Challenges are a good sign. Welcome challenges because they show you're ready. You are a badass for being here. You're a badass for attracting these challenges. You're a badass when you get through them, and you're a badass during them.

And if you're thinking you didn't sign up for this, well, that's an interesting topic. Have you ever seen those memes you see on Instagram, saying, 'Stop the world, I'm getting off' or 'I didn't sign up for this'? As far as I'm concerned, that attitude is bonkers, because none of us signed up for this and none of us is exempt from challenges. We all have challenges on different levels. We all have the same fears, we just have different tools to overcome them. Your soul may be up there saying, "This is exactly the lesson your human needs to get. And this is exactly what's supposed to happen." As a human, it feels like you didn't sign up for it, but on a soul level, it's about our evolution.

Remember that self-love makes the recovery from challenges shorter, but it doesn't remove the challenges altogether. If some challenges take a little time to naff-off out of your life as you shift to a next level and become a manifesting queen, know that there's a divine plan and it's all laid out perfectly. The lessons you're supposed to learn are coming to you in the perfect time and all for your greatest good.

PS Here's Your Self-Love Medicine

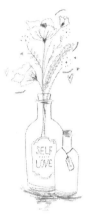

Clear space for self-love and goodness in your life, starting with forgiveness!

I am yet to forgive myself for...

Things that get in the way of self-love and are no longer serving me in my life are...

Thought patterns...

Relationships...

Foods...

Drinks...

Habits...

Places...

Behaviours...

Belongings...

CHAPTER THREE

Trusting Me, Trusting You

"The healer you have been looking for
is your own courage to know and love
yourself completely."

Yung Pueblo

Would you love someone you didn't trust? If a person is unpredictable, it makes it tricky to trust them and even harder to love them. What about when that person is yourself? Self-love is about learning to trust that you are always doing your best and cultivating faith that everything is working out for your highest good.

In this step, we'll look at how you can achieve self-trust through honing your intuition and strengthening your inner GPS.

When you trust, you show up in the world differently and manifest from that place. You can fuck up 1,000 times and know that you still deserve love. However, a lack of self-trust can take you away from feeling love towards yourself. It can increase self-doubt and

Choices are how you
vote for your own vision.

PS I Love Me
www.ginaswire.com

make you feel a desire for constant acknowledgement. Lack of trust also stokes indecision, perfectionism and a fear of failure.

On the other hand, trusting the process and trusting yourself is a pathway to loving yourself more. It is something you can do for yourself and something you can build. It helps you to set realistic goals and then, when you achieve them, it expands your self-confidence, makes it easier to make decisions and reduces stress levels. Trusting yourself also helps others to trust you, which can lead to great things.

It takes deep intuition to reach this place of trust. Without this, you might be lost, lacking confidence and feeling unsure. But once you master it, you will absolutely soar, because it means you can stop relying on other people's opinions and tune in to your own wisdom.

What is intuition?

My definition of intuition is that it is a kind of collective intelligence or collective consciousness that we, as individuals, can *feel* inside ourselves. We can experience this as an inner voice, body wisdom, heart wisdom, personal wisdom, a 'sense', a 'gut feeling' or a 'knowing'.

Do you ever feel like there's a place within you that 'just knows'? That's because intuition doesn't come from the mind. It comes from somewhere else. It is a deep, deep sense of knowing that we can tap into anytime. We can ask that place within for answers, because all the answers are already inside us. The saying that *We have everything we need already within ourselves* is completely true, even though it often doesn't feel like it. In that way, intuition is like self-love. It is not something we need to *gain* or learn *how* to have. It is our natural state. It's just that we can forget our natural state when we start over-analysing or when our conditioning becomes louder than our inner voice.

Intuition is always there, but often we can't hear it and need to remove the shit that prevents us from hearing our own voice. Many people resist this notion, thinking they don't hear anything and don't have any signs of which direction to take, but that's not the case. It's simply that we block our intuition with the mind. Intuition is not thinking. Intuition is a feeling sense. What often happens is that we start *thinking* instead of *feeling*, creating confusion and resistance.

The aim is to think less. Whenever we don't know the answer to something or are faced with indecision, we need to stop thinking about it. This may sound counterintuitive, but letting the mind wander is key to letting our intuition do its job. Sometimes the best thing we can do is to just 'sleep on it' because we'll have the answer by the morning. This is a perfect example of intuition, because when you give your mind a rest from thinking, the inner knowing can come to the surface. Even just going for a walk in nature can allow your mind to wander and give it enough space for the answer to come.

Why we need intuition

> "No problem can be solved from the same level of consciousness that created it."
> Albert Einstein

Why is intuition so important? When we tap into intuition, we can rely on ourselves more. When we trust ourselves, we show up. When we show up in the world, we manifest more trust. Compare for a moment how somebody behaves when they don't trust, when they are constantly questioning their trust in their partner, their job, their client, themselves. They show up with a different energy, one where they're uncertain. On the other hand, when somebody is in full trust, knowing that whatever happens, happens, they just go for it. They behave differently, they are self-reliant and they own their power.

So often, our go-to can become relying on other people and their opinions. I used to do this too. I would run everything by my mum because I didn't trust myself. It can be helpful to ask for help from others and see what other people think, but the problem arises when we outsource our power and give away ownership of our needs and desires. When we do this, we weaken our own wisdom by believing we don't really know what's best for ourselves.

You *do* know what is best for you, even if you've lost touch with it. Your intuition brought you here.

Tapping into intuition

Fortunately, self-trust is something that we can practise, by honing our intuition and learning to have more confidence in it. Knowing yourself and trusting yourself strengthens self-love. We can build self-trust by using a simple but powerful question. I call it the 'Golden Question':

Does this feel right?

This question helps you to tap into what you already know to be true. It creates space for your inner knowing to communicate what feels right. You could use any example or any situation that you're weighing up. Which option do you *feel* is more right for you? Not which seems safer, more logical or more practical, but which *feels right*?

There are other ways to practise too. When you wake up in the morning, before speaking to your mum, dad, cats, partner or friend, before you check your phone, before you do all the things, I invite you to ask yourself:

How do I feel today? What do I need?

See what comes through. It is quick and simple to ask yourself. You can still involve others in your decision, but at least you've asked yourself and checked in with your own intuition first.

Once you have started noticing how you feel, there are some practical ways to tap into your intuition actively. Here are some options for you to try:

- Permission slips

- Muscle testing

- Pendulums

- Tossing a coin

- Asking for a sign

- Tuning in to body sensations

- Rehearsing your options

Let me walk you through some of my favourites!

Permission

On some occasions, it is not that our intuition isn't pointing towards something, but that we haven't given ourselves permission to do something, and so we are refusing to hear our inner voice. A 'permission slip' means granting yourself the permission to do something.

This worked successfully with one of my clients. She had been told that she would make a fantastic singer, something she had always wanted to do. However, she had not given herself permission to go and do that. As part of her coaching, I gave her a written permission slip to do it. When she felt she had permission, she decided to go and give it a try.

Giving yourself a permission slip allows you to relax and trust what you already know, removing any ideas that you aren't allowed.

Body wisdom

You may have heard of muscle testing, a method of using your body's wisdom to find your 'yes' and your 'no' through the way your body reacts to questioning. The easiest way to tap into this is by using a pendulum, which is a stone/crystal on the end of a cord/chain which you suspend from your thumb and forefinger. When you ask a question, it will indicate an answer by spinning one way or another. Unlike what some people may think, it is not the crystal that holds the wisdom; it's you and your body's energy.

Gut feeling

Figuring out your gut feeling can be so much simpler than you may think. Remember when, as a child, you would toss a coin to make a choice? We may have been using it for trivial decisions at the time, but even if you have a big decision to make, flipping a coin can help you with indecision.

Immediately, your reaction speaks volumes!

If you get a feeling of relief when the coin lands, that's a sign it's right. And if the coin lands and you feel disappointment, that's a sign that the opposite is true for you. Just like the pendulum, it's not the coin that makes the decision, but the feeling you get.

Keeping with the coin analogy, there's also this idea of cosmic coins. Fear and trust are two sides of the same coin. You can't fear something if you fully trust it. And you can't trust something if you fear it. The cosmic coin concept means you can choose either trust or fear at any point, but you can only choose one. So, which do you choose? Is it trust or is it fear?

Signs

Another way you might tap into intuition is by simply asking for a sign. It's an age-old way of tapping into intuition.

I'll ask for a sign and I'll just know when I see it. For example, I wasn't sure if I should fly from LA to Bali or LA to the UK, so I surrendered and asked for a sign. The next moment, I saw a mini painted Union Jack flag. Boom! There's my sign. Another example is what my great friend and client, Kim, does, which is asking to see blue owls when she's on track. Specific, I know! But when we were walking through the streets of Ibiza after she had a hugely transformational retreat, there they were... ceramic blue owls, loads of them. We get signs all the time. Look out for them. Ask and then notice what is there!

Body sensations

Have you ever been asked on a date and when the guy says he wants to see you again, your body shrinks down? Contraction is a sign that it's a no. Or have you been in conversation and suddenly got goose pimples on your arms? Some people say that goose pimples indicate the presence of truth or that something is right for them. These are examples of your body *signalling* something to you.

I had a huge realisation that there was a big piece of clearing I needed to do in my life. As soon as I thought it, I got full-body goose pimples and for about five minutes after. I take that as a clear sign that I'm in my truth. Likewise, when I'm on a call with a client and we get to the bottom of something that has been plaguing their life for a long time, sometimes up to 20 or 30 years, my body responds. I always show them my forearm hairs standing on end and tell them what that means. Cool, isn't it?

Your body *knows*. Looking out for its reactions and noticing what it is telling you can be a great way of tapping into your intuition. Rather than asking your mind, ask your body, ask your heart, ask your gut.

Rehearse your options

Another technique for tapping into intuition is taking your options for a test drive. Here's how you do that:

1. Ask the question. Make sure it's specific and clear. Check in to see if you are resisting making the decision. Is this something you don't want to decide?

2. Notice any self-talk and notice if you truly want this. Sometimes it's not your own desire but someone else's that you're acting on. Maybe your friends want you to go somewhere and you're doing it for them, or maybe something is a good idea, but it's not the right timing for you. Tune into that.

3. Rehearse the options in your mind and 'try them on'. Ask yourself the Golden Question. Does this feel right?

And if you don't know, you can always sleep on it!

Trust always works

"When you learn that you can trust life, life will deliver treasures beyond your imagination."
Debbie Ford

By now, it should be clear why we need trust, but have you ever considered who you are trusting? We trust in ourselves. We trust in the world. We trust in our body. We trust in humanity. We trust in our innate wisdom. And by trusting our intuition, we're trusting collective intelligence.

Trusting is also self-love, because as I mentioned earlier, when you trust, you show up in the world differently and good things manifest from that place. Trust breeds confidence, love, peace and joy, so when we go out into the world feeling these higher-frequency states, we attract higher-frequency people, opportunities and abundance. When you trust that the Universe is conspiring to help you have the most amazing life and help as many other people as possible along the way, it feels like everything is rigged in your favour. In fact, believing that *everything is rigged in your favour* can help you have the attitude that makes it so. If I am out of trust one day, I may feel scarcity, lack, anxiety, fear, sadness or overwhelm. And if I feel this, it's like I am invisible in the world.

Like with self-love, where it's easy to love yourself when it's going well, but more difficult when shit hits the fan, it's easier to feel trust when things are going well than when they're going badly. Yet, having trust implicitly means that we can still believe that everything is working out the way it is supposed to, even when things are challenging. What is important to remember is that trust creates expansion. Fear contracts. Trust expands.

Let's use relationships as an example. When you're with someone in a relationship, you've got two choices: to trust or not to trust. If you don't trust, everything's going to be restricted, strained, strangled. As soon as you start to trust, you feel it opening, opening, opening. That's not to say things won't go wrong or your path won't change. When I look back on things that 'went wrong' for me in the past, I think maybe it went just right. Maybe it was a cosmic get-out-of-jail-free card!

It's only when we start to source our worthiness from *within* that we can truly understand our power,

become magnetic

and attract what we want.

PS I Love Me
www.ginaswire.com

Interestingly, statistics show that somebody who isn't trusted is more likely to cheat than someone who is trusted, which means that the unwanted situation is manifesting by being non-trusting. Being in a state of distrust or worry is almost like praying over and over for something you don't want.

When have you trusted yourself and it turned out to be right?

For me, it was the tug to travel to India and learn more about self-love. I was at home in Manchester, and I kept hearing a guided whisper... *Go to India.* I didn't understand it at first, but I had a sense I should go, even though it had never been on my radar. I began to notice signs, which I saw everywhere: it would be mentioned on TV, I'd see pictures in magazines, I bought items and would see on the labels 'Made in India'. I started really paying attention and eventually trusted this feeling inside that I had to go there.

After the yoga teacher training that I was booked on, I had planned to travel with some friends from the course. But the day we were supposed to leave, something didn't feel right. I felt guided again... *Don't go to Hampi.* But I couldn't understand it. After all, the tickets were already booked and what else was I supposed to do? That morning, as I was getting ready to leave, a place became available on an advanced yoga teacher training course. As soon as I heard, it was a 'heaven, yes'. I signed up and knew straight away that it was right.

A month later, I understood why. Towards the end of the course, I found out why my inner GPS had taken me to India and urged me to stay for the advanced teacher training instead of heading off with my friends. I met an amazing man and fell in love for the first time.

Divine timing and inner guidance had put me in a place that I'd never have been if it wasn't for trust.

Creating our own reality

When, in your life, have you trusted yourself and you were 'wrong' but good has come out of it or something happened that needed to happen? Even though something may suck at the time, you can remain committed to yourself and actively trust your healing. This does not mean bypassing challenging feelings, but it can mean reaching harmony more quickly. The time it takes to acknowledge and accept what happens is shorter when we trust that everything is taking us where we need to go to learn the lessons we need to learn. This brings us a fuller, richer life experience.

Why do our souls make our human selves have these challenges in our lives? The answer can be a little confronting, but also powerful. We create our own reality. Our souls want these experiences for us, want us to meet certain people or take certain directions. Our souls are guiding us and it's about trusting that the experience is for our evolution. Our souls know exactly what they are doing and don't need answers. Our human selves feel like we need answers, but if we can just trust that there's a plan and it's divine, we can trust the timing of our lives.

PS I Love Me Practice

Here is a fantastic exercise to dive into if you're curious about why you've chosen a particular reality. You can do this whenever you experience something that you didn't want to attract or when something feels like it's going 'wrong'.

1. Take a deep breath and get still. Now, say to yourself:

   I'm creating this for myself. I wonder why that is?

   Why was I a match for this situation?

2. See what comes up.

   Example: Let's say someone cheated on you in a relationship. You might realise you were cheating yourself the entire time.

When something happens and you can't figure out why, this exercise can be a fun way to explore other ways to look at it and avoid falling for the disempowering question: "Why is this happening to me?"

PS I Love Me Practice

Likewise, you can channel a little wisdom when making a decision.

1. Imagine someone whose actions inspire you.

2. Whether it's grandmother energy, the most successful person in your field or an entrepreneur, ask how they would act in your situation.

    Examples: What would my grandmother do? What would Beyoncé do? What would Richard Branson do? These are some that I like to use.

3. Now imagine what they would do.

Alternative technique:

1. Visualise what you would do if someone gave you a million pounds/dollars. Use your imagination and just see what comes through, and then see if that helps inspire your decision.

    Example: If someone gave me a million pounds, the first thing I would do is create experiences to help people through my business: a retreat centre in Portugal on a hill with sea views and self-love teacher trainings.

However you tap into your intuition, know that you can trust how it is all working out and that you are creating your own reality.

PS Here's Your Self-Love Medicine

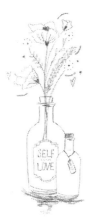

What would you do if you trusted it was all working out? If you just knew 100% that everything you desired was about to happen, how would you think, act and be this week?

CHAPTER FOUR

Trigger Happy

"You're the narrator, the protagonist and the sidekick. You're the storyteller and the story told. You are somebody's something, but you are also your you."

John Green

In any relationship you ever have, getting to know someone more deeply and understanding how they think and feel is always going to create more space for love, connection and empathy. Getting to know *yourself* is exactly the same. The more you know yourself, the more you can love yourself naturally.

When you get to know yourself deeply, things will come up that you'll need to examine and understand. In particular, sometimes we have an emotional response to what's happening to us in the present moment that reminds us of something in our past. Unexamined, this can have a huge impact on what we decide to do next and the way we behave, meaning we can get stuck in a pattern that does us no good.

Self-love

makes the recovery from
challenges shorter.

In this fourth step to your self-love transformation, we're going to dive into what triggers our emotional responses, and how we keep ourselves stuck and unable to move forward.

Self-love vocabulary

I'll be introducing a few concepts in this chapter, so before we start, here's a little run-down of what the words mean:

Trigger – an emotional response to something in the present moment that relates to or reminds you of a past experience (when you get curious about what it really is)

Block – a perceived inability to move forward with something or reach a goal, as in 'writer's block'

Limiting belief – an ineffective thought pattern that you've been thinking for so long you accept it as truth

Story – a narrative that you keep telling yourself or others to explain what happened in your experience or justify your emotions

Pattern – when you keep thinking, doing or behaving the same way over and over, sometimes in different situations, even if it doesn't serve you.

All of these create opportunities for self-love. If you avoid looking at them, you cut yourself off from knowing yourself better and deepening your self-love.

You have to feel it to heal it

The only way to heal yourself is to fully feel your emotions. You can't bypass your feelings and be fully loving and accepting of yourself. You have to go into them and through them to reach the other side. Triggers are the gateway to accessing those emotions.

I'll give you an example of a time when I used my triggers to access something about myself that I needed to know in order to be more fully self-accepting and self-loving. I was on my way to an event in Bali and a few things happened in succession that all made me feel triggered. Even knowing logically that they were happening for good reason, in the moment, it still sucked.

First, I bumped into my ex-boyfriend and his new girlfriend. Even though it was a mutual breakup, or 'conscious uncoupling' as they say in my community in Bali, the interaction still triggered me. In other words, I had an emotional response. When I stopped and tuned in, I felt *unchosen*, even though that wasn't the circumstance at all.

Then, I was having some wonderful conversations with a gorgeous, exciting man, whom I'd met at the event. We hung out together and arranged to meet up, but later on I saw him sensually massaging another girl and again I felt triggered. I assessed what was going on inside and it was the same trigger: not feeling *chosen*.

And then some friends of mine decided to meet up with other people and not invite me. Again, I was feeling all the *unchosen* feels.

After a few repeated triggers, I got the message. I knew I needed to feel this pain to move through it. So, I felt more deeply into what these experiences reminded me of. In my conscious adult mind, I knew it didn't make sense, but my inner little girl was still wounded and wanted to be chosen and needed. She was worried about being abandoned again, just like I had felt when I was small. That little girl was running the show (awwwwww! Cuteness overload!).

Once I made this connection, everything changed. In my conscious mind, I realised I can never be abandoned again. I am already chosen, as I choose myself. I don't need a man to choose me to feel or be worthy of love. I can self-source all the love and worthiness from within. Love is infinite and knowing this is the gift of my trigger. Thank you, trigger!

Trigger 0, Gina 1.

If we go through life feeling these intense feelings, but not understanding what triggers them, or how to move through them, we are unable to heal. This causes persistent blocks that prevent you from achieving your goals and moving forward with your life.

Exploring your triggers

When someone says or does something and you have an instant and intense emotional response, we call it a trigger. Triggers are not inherently bad. In fact, they can be incredibly helpful, because they help identify stories from the past that are blocking you and making you feel stuck.

As an example, let's say your partner says you didn't do something that you were supposed to do. An immediate reaction could be frustration, "Oh my God, why is he even talking about that?" You could be up in your head straight away and respond defensively or end up in an argument. Another emotion that may be triggered is sadness, with thoughts such as, "Why is he saying that to me? What have I done wrong? Nothing I do is ever good enough."

Being 'in your head' means it's no longer about the event or conversation that's happening now. It's no longer about you. It's no longer about your partner. The interaction has triggered an emotional response that reminds you of something that has happened in the past. A trigger is never about what is in front of you; it's always about the past story.

So, before we go any further, I'd like you to identify some triggers of your own and keep them in mind as you go through this chapter. Often, we blame our triggered reactions on being hungry, tired or hormonal, but we know that's a bit of a cop out, right? When we look beneath the trigger and the behaviour, it is usually showing us something that could be *healed*.

PS I Love Me Practice

In this exercise, we're going to turn your triggers into your teachers! This one is all about learning how to follow that thread back through your past experiences and know more about yourself, accept what happened, and move forward.

1. First, identify a trigger.

    When have you been triggered lately?

    What do you notice about the thoughts that come up?

    What do you notice about the reaction you had?

    Take a moment to write down anything that comes up.

    Example: I asked my partner to pick up some soup from the shop, but he came back with the wrong one. I felt angry at him and said, "You said you were going to get a different one and now I've ended up with a soup that I can't eat." I started thinking about how I didn't have the right food to eat and how I didn't like what he had bought me. These thoughts set off feelings of resentment.

2. Next, get curious and ask yourself some juicy questions.

    What is this really about?

    What is coming up for me?

How do I feel about this? Let down? Pissed off? Embarrassed?

What does it remind me of?

Example: I realised I was feeling a bit let down because my needs were not met by my partner when he came home with the wrong soup. What this was really about was feeling let down. Which reminded me of when Dad said he was going to pick me up from school, but he wasn't there.

3. Look at other times you have experienced this before.

   Why is this a familiar dynamic or pattern?

   Who did you become when you were interacting with this person in this situation?

   Who did the other person become in the situation?

   Example: My partner reminded me of Dad when he picked me up late and just brushed off the fact that he wasn't there and didn't apologise. In this situation, I reacted just like I did that day when Dad let me down.

4. Identify where healing needs to happen.

   Example: Perhaps it wasn't Dad's fault that he was late that day, but that little girl who got left at school pick-up still needs a hug.

Our triggers become our teachers, so instead of labelling your triggers as 'wrong' when you're emotionally triggered by something, get *curious* and ask yourself what it's really about and why.

Doing the opposite

Once you know what needs to be healed or what the so-called 'block' may be, how do you get unstuck from your familiar dynamics or patterns? Have you ever tried simply doing the opposite? It sounds almost too simple, doesn't it? But hear me out.

On one of my retreats, there was a woman who had been in a relationship for 30 years. The relationship had served her quite well until the last 10 years, when she had started questioning whether it was still right for her, and whether she should stay or leave. She was so caught up in indecision that it had become a block which affected all areas of her life. I suggested simply *doing the opposite.*

I got her to imagine that there was no decision to make for a whole day, a whole week, a whole month, the rest of her life. If there was no decision to be made, how would she live her life? Framing it like this, she was able to take the decision off the table and become present to the reality of her life as it really was, rather than constantly living in a negative future fantasy. Lo and behold, this act of trust and surrender – shaken and stirred with a shot of Universal magic – meant she was able to harmonise her relationship with herself. And much to her own amazement and everyone else's on the retreat, she started to enjoy her partner's company again! She was stunned and a bit flummoxed when she reported this in our post retreat WhatsApp thread. And this, ladies, is how we roll in the self-love vortex.

Simply *doing the opposite* can be an effective strategy when we feel blocked, because when we take the 'stuck' feeling out of the equation, our *resistance* to making a decision dissolves, and we are able to live our life fully. What if we don't need to make a decision? What if we're just not meant to know the answer right now? We're all so used to looking, searching and desperately wanting to be certain of what lies ahead. But if we can begin to trust in the divine timing of our life, we can start to trust that these patterns, cycles and triggers are there for a reason: to teach us something. In divine time, you'll get the answers you need.

For years, I'd been working with the trigger of abandonment, which would come up in many different ways, because of my childhood story of my father leaving and going to a new family. Any time I had a heated discussion with my then boyfriend, he would withstand it for a while, but then he would get annoyed and leave, slamming the door on his way out and turning off his phone so I couldn't contact him. His disappearance would trigger me because I felt abandoned that he had left. It didn't matter in that moment that I was a totally independent woman who has travelled around the world on her own and who could look after her own emotional needs. The trigger was automatically *abandonment*. Abandonment was what felt real. By barking up the abandonment tree for so long, I was stuck in that same story, affirming and ingraining it even more deeply.

When I was able to take a step back and become the observer of the trigger, I could lovingly hold space for my inner child which allowed me to recognise that the opposite was true – that with self-love I would never be abandoned again. Because I now know that I've got my inner mother, healer, lover and best friend with me at all times. Yey!

To assist you in transcending the loop of hell that triggers catapult us headfirst into, *doing the opposite* can be the welcome healer you've been praying for.

If, when you get triggered, you normally get caught up in anger and rage, it might be healing for you to take a moment, ask for a time out, pop yourself in a room, light a candle, listen to some whale sounds/Enya/Moby (whatever floats your cosmic slow boat) and practise breathing like a pro. Or, if you're like me and prone to a freeze/appease response, which can lead to supressing your truth and never speaking up for yourself, it's an absolute gift to the system to organise a rage ritual. This could mean consciously and safely screaming into your hands or a cushion, pummelling your bed or pillow fights with your teddy bears!!!

For a breathwork practice and an anger release playlist, head to www.ginaswire.com/bookresources.

Is that a fact?

Another way of challenging a belief that underlies a trigger is to ask the question:

Is that a fact?

The reason this question works is because being stuck is a *perception*. Usually stories, patterns and limiting beliefs appear as blocks or something holding you back, which you identify using triggers that are more obvious, surface level and easy to spot.

When you examine a belief, there is nothing physical in your way. There is no real reason you can't do something. It is not a fact, not a tangible block to your progress.

Asking this question switches you out of your head and puts you into the present moment. It takes you out of the past stories, patterns or limiting beliefs that are being triggered, and puts you into the truth of the here and now, which is the best place to be, because it stops you from being limited by things that might have been facts in the past but are now behind you.

When you spot a trigger and identify the underlying block, it is common to use it as an excuse not to take action. So, the question to ask next is this:

Your intuition
brought you here.

PS I Love Me
www.ginaswire.com

Do I really want it?

Do you really want the end goal? Are you hiding behind a block as an excuse? Often, if we say we are blocked, then we don't even try and we act like it doesn't matter if we fail. When we take this approach, failure is almost inevitable because we let ourselves get triggered over and over, and we allow our perception to determine our action or inaction.

This means it's really important to use those triggers to determine what stories or limiting beliefs are at play, so we can stop using them as reasons not to go after what we truly want. Remember, going after what you truly want is a sign of self-love, so this is about eliminating what's standing in the way of that.

Stories evolve...

Over time, if you don't deal with your triggers, you will tell your stories over and over until they become your firm beliefs. This is because when you tell a story, to yourself or to someone else, you are recreating it. Then the next time a situation comes up, you access the memory of the last time you told the story, not the original story. The story you are telling eventually isn't the same as the original. It evolves as it gets retold. In other words, you find a story to fit the new situation in front of you and make a story fit the point you are trying to make. It's not lying. It's editing. And it's a natural human trait. Humans are highly intelligent and change our stories to match our environment.

Eventually, we believe our own narrative, but is it the ultimate truth? Well, it's not necessarily the original story or the truth, but it's also not necessarily false, because by believing in our stories, we can act in a way that it becomes our truth. It's important to remember that there's always another way and that you can change your story by finding another perspective.

When I was a plus-size model, I was often told I wasn't quite big enough for my clients and they would sometimes ask that I gain weight to get the job or pad my body, so I looked bigger. They would choose images that were taken from an unflattering angle. Sometimes, the first time I would see the image was in a magazine or on a billboard, which, for a 20-something woman with street cred to think about, was traumatic. Meanwhile, in my personal life, I was two dress sizes bigger than all my friends, and in that part of my life, it was all about being smaller. One guy even said he would date me if I could get down to a size 10! (I mean... *what?!*) Of course, it was the exact same body that everyone was looking at, but I was too big for some and too small for others.

See? It's often about how we view a situation. Nobody is strictly 'wrong' here. Everyone just held a different view of the same thing. All versions can be true. It's not right and it's not wrong. It's whatever we perceive it to be. In the end, none of your blocks are true. It's all smoke and mirrors, stories and perspectives. Every belief is human-made, and every story is changeable.

PS I Love Me Practice

You can practise changing your perception of any situation, seeing the story from the other side, by getting into the habit of asking that all-important question.

1. In the moment, notice your thought.

2. Ask yourself:

   Is that a fact?

3. Be a natural, neutral observer. Listen and see what's there to expand your awareness.

And you can notice it in other people too, being curious when they are questioning themselves, and recognising what beliefs seem to be limiting them. (Important! You can notice but try not to mention it to them or judge. This is an exercise in becoming aware of different perspectives, not about becoming that annoying person who gives others uninvited feedback!)

Exploring your triggers and blocks increases your self-awareness, which grows your capacity to love. The more you know yourself, the more you can love yourself, and this is the pathway to being, getting and having what you want in your life.

PS Here's Your Self-Love Medicine

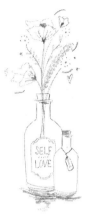

Before you move on to the next chapter, look back to the trigger you wrote down at the beginning of this chapter.

How has your perspective shifted? How do you feel about the issue now?

Using your new awareness from this chapter, look at where you've felt triggered or blocked recently.

What is the trigger really about? What feelings are you avoiding by staying blocked?

Write down your thoughts.

CHAPTER FIVE

It's Been Emotional (And The Future Will Be Too)

"Depression, pain and fear are gifts that say, 'Sweetheart, take a look at your thinking right now. You're living in a story that isn't true for you'."

Byron Katie

E motion or *e-motion* is said to be energy in motion. Any emotional state is energy moving. Emotions aren't inherently 'good' or 'bad', except when we attach meaning to them, but they can be useful in directing us in our life.

For deep self-love to exist you must understand all of your emotions and accept that they are part of the human experience, so emotional intelligence is something of a prerequisite. Without this understanding you won't know what you are numbing, avoiding or suppressing. As Brené Brown says in *The Gifts of Imperfection*, "We cannot selectively numb emotions. When we numb the painful emotions, we also numb the positive emotions."

When you trust that the
Universe is conspiring to help
you have *the most amazing life,*
and help as many other people
as possible along the way,
it feels like *everything is
rigged in your favour!*

Step five of the self-love transformation is about becoming more intelligent in your emotional life and how to move from being numbed-out to fully accepting all that is there.

Emotional intelligence

Emotional intelligence, or having a high emotional quotient (EQ), means understanding emotions and what they are trying to tell us. In other words, emotional intelligence is knowing yourself emotionally, being able to ask yourself what you are feeling and recognising the emotion quickly. Emotional intelligence is not just useful in knowing yourself and your own emotions, but it also gives you the ability to use that intelligence to relate to other people, to relate to yourself, and to ask for what you want. When you start getting good at recognising what is going on in yourself, you will, by default, become good at recognising other people's emotional states. This can be helpful with friends, family, children, colleagues, everyone around you. It cultivates compassion for others because you've experienced what they're feeling. You can only truly understand an emotion in someone else that you've felt yourself.

Emotional intelligence is knowing that there's always a whole host of emotions going on inside us. Emotions don't just happen at peak moments, like having a baby or winning a lottery. There are many more emotions that we feel all the time. The more you feel the light *and* the dark, the more you can experience. And the more you have ups and downs in your life, the more emotionally intelligent, empathetic and compassionate you become.

When we struggle to identify our emotions, we can start to attach a story to what is going on in front of us. We often become reactive or behave in problematic ways. Taking a few steps back, taking a breath and recognising what we're dealing with in an emotionally intelligent way is something we can practise to move forward in our lives more consciously.

PS I Love Me Practice

Being able to name your emotions and even where they are in your body has real benefits for becoming more in tune with your own emotions and others'.

1. Notice the sensations in your body. Perhaps you identify a heavy feeling in your heart, or you feel unstable or shaky at the base of your spine.

2. Give those sensations a voice by naming them out loud. Even if you have a real mixture of feelings in the body and can't figure out what any of them are, you can voice that confusion: "There is confusion."

Numbing

There are so many emotions going on at any one time. As humans, we have a lot to deal with, don't we? There are so many things going on in our lives and often we don't know how to handle everything happening inside of us. We can feel alone in dealing with our emotions and the discomfort can feel intense. And what do we do when our emotions get too much? We numb them out.

We might not realise we are doing this at the time, but most of us can relate to wanting a glass of wine after a stressful day at work. We have all numbed our emotions at some point and we do this in different ways – shopping, eating, drinking, partying, drugs, gambling, sex, keeping busy, and other distractions like TV or our own drama. Even personal development or going to the gym can be used to numb out, because numbing is anything excessive. It doesn't have to be 'bad for you' to be bad for you.

Sometimes these things can be medicine if they are done consciously. However, often they are used to suppress the stress. In other words, we do them when we have an emotional trigger that we can't fully understand, heal, embrace or accept. Rather than being uncomfortable, we turn to these things to numb the emotion or change our state of mind.

The consequence of deliberately numbing the uncomfortable emotions is that we numb the ones we want to feel too. Whenever I used to watch a sad movie, I would never, ever cry because I had fixed myself with the identity that I was a strong independent woman. I might feel a lump in my throat, but I would hold it all in. The thing is, I wasn't only refusing to feel sadness by doing this, I was not allowing myself to feel love, to feel free. Sure, I was numbing feelings of powerlessness, but that stopped me from feeling powerful. I never felt heartbreak, but equally, I never fell in love. I never felt dread or upset, and I used to think I'd cracked it, always living between good and great. Especially when my friends would experience the kind of absolute heartbreak that follows the end of true love. When they couldn't get out of bed I would think, "I don't want that. I'm winning right where I am. I like living between good and great."

It's impossible to feel the highs without also feeling the lows. Numbing protects us from what we're scared of feeling, but if we're frightened of being abandoned, cheated on or rejected and dull those sensations, we will be unable to open to being deeply in love.

PS I Love Me Practice

In this exercise, I'm going to ask you a bunch of questions so that you can get to know yourself more and make some big positive changes.

1. Take as long as you like to close your eyes and answer these questions.

   Is there anything you're numbing?

   Are there any emotions that you don't allow yourself to feel or feel fully?

   If you don't allow yourself to feel, how else do you cope? Do you party? Shop? Constantly make sure you're busy? Avoid being alone so you don't have to feel your feelings?

2. Take out a pen and paper and write down anything that comes to mind. It may not make a lot of sense. Just put pen to paper and see what comes out. Take a look at your answers and make sure you've been really honest with yourself. There is huge potential to grow when you open up to feeling what you don't want to feel.

3. Stay with this heightened state of awareness now for the next few weeks and notice where you would normally numb yourself.

When this comes up, instead of going to your default behaviour, close your eyes, breathe and repeat the affirmation: *It's safe for me to feel.*

Allow the feeling to prevail and stay with it. You will notice that the feeling passes naturally without the need to numb it. This can take some practice at first, but trust me when I say it's the path to self-love.

Connecting with your emotions

How can you build your EQ further and begin to understand this cocktail of emotions? Here are a few suggestions:

- Taking a few breaths is so simple and effective. It puts you in the present moment and sends a signal to your body to relax and feel safe.

- Stopping to notice what is here now enables you to instantly disengage from future-focused worrying, allowing you to feel what's really happening inside of you.

- Journalling is probably my most recommended hack for self-love; it's a free, safe space for you to allow anything and everything and see it for what it is.

- Meditation has been proven to increase self-awareness, EQ and self-love.

- Connecting with your body, and noticing the subtle sensations that are always there, helps you to access your emotions as they are stored in the body rather than the head (dancing or walking in nature are great ways to connect to your body, or scanning your body from the top of your head to the tips of your toes and seeing what you can feel without any judgment).

- Hire a coach or mentor. A skilful coach can help you open up your blind spots and help you develop EQ faster than you could do alone.

Incorporating some of these practices into your life will expand your capacity to be present to what *is* and love yourself more.

If you're feeling disconnected from yourself and your emotional state, reconnection is everything. When you can, reconnect to the feelings in your body, drop into what these emotions are. Let them move through you without attaching to them. Being there for yourself, holding space for yourself, listening to yourself, tuning in, giving yourself quality time, letting yourself repair and recoup your energy, letting your cup refill, this is where a connection to yourself starts.

When you foster this connection with yourself, you can expect a deeper connection with other people too. Here's why. Think of when you ask someone how they are. Someone who isn't in touch with their emotions might reply, "I'm fine." People do this all the time, but it shows a lack of care. It's shutting the door in the face of the person asking. Someone who is in touch with their emotions might reply, "Hmm, I'm fine, but I'm having some challenges, and I'm feeling a little bit lost and a bit betrayed. I'm feeling okay, but it's a little bit weird at the moment, and I'm just using all my self-care practices to help myself." This reply might astonish the person receiving it because of its vulnerability, its openness, its emotional intelligence and its willingness to be human. And that honesty fosters respect and connection. It brings us together as humans.

Connecting to our emotional intelligence leads to creating deeper relationships; partnerships, friendships, family relationships, client relationships, business relationships and more, because when we become more emotionally intelligent, we're able to gauge how others are feeling and anticipate their needs. We are also able to ask for what we want in a way that others will really understand. Getting what you want is part of self-love, and most people don't know how to ask for that in a loving, effective way because they don't know how to express themselves. By expanding your EQ, you are on the way to understanding what you want, being confident enough to ask for it and skilful enough to get it.

Susan, a client of mine in New York, had been having a lot of friction with her husband. A few days after we started working on EQ, she messaged me, "Wow, Gina, I can't believe what has happened!" She had managed to have a deep and meaningful conversation with her husband – finally – and he had spoken his truth for the first time ever and she felt heard by him. After that, their sex life massively improved, and she ended up falling pregnant. Falling out of love with herself, her body and her husband, because she couldn't get pregnant, had been the original reason she had come to me for help.

Start to use your EQ in your everyday life: when you're alone, talking with your friends and family or at work. By following the steps above each day, you are likely to start manifesting better outcomes, getting more opportunities, receiving more and giving more, because there's more to give.

EQ is the future

Emotional intelligence is not just incredibly useful on a personal level, but it is a wonderful way to close deals and create relatability, which is why huge corporations like Google and Uber train their staff in emotional intelligence.

Julie, a client of mine, worked in a job she loved but felt undervalued by her boss. She had spoken to him before and hadn't had a good response at all. She felt fobbed off. After working with me, she explained to her boss boldly and lovingly what she needed and why she needed it, in a way that he would not be defensive towards her. She ended up leaving that meeting with a 30% pay rise and a new sense of empowerment for asking for what she wanted in a new way, using the EQ concepts I'd taught her.

In life, we are always 'pitching', and emotional intelligence is key to getting things to happen. Using your emotional intelligence, you tackle situations differently depending on what you're picking up. For instance, let's say you're asking a friend to lunch (a 'pitch' of sorts). You might realise that one friend who loves being in the limelight would respond better to something like, "Hey, do you want to go to that fancy place we've been meaning to try and get stuck into some high-vibe conversations?" While another more introverted friend might prefer, "Hey, would you like to chill over a bite to eat?" What we want is not much different between the two, but the way we pitch it using our own emotional intelligence can help us get more of what we want and give more of what other people want. It's a win-win situation.

This pitch for lunch is a minor example, but you can apply the exact same principle for navigating bigger life situations, such as romantic challenges or career obstacles. Every relationship benefits from a little injection of EQ.

Emotional intelligence is the future for other reasons too. Creativity and emotional intelligence will be the most in-demand skills in the future workforce, as these qualities cannot be replaced by machines. Emotional intelligence makes us more adaptable, compassionate, likeable, trustworthy and authentic. It also makes us better conversationalists. It's an intelligence unlike the kind we were measured on in school. That kind of intelligence is not only dry and linear, but also replicable. Can you tell I was the kid at school who was holding regular 'agony aunt' sessions at lunchtime, and getting messages from the Universe even then? The school I went to back then had no way of recognising or 'marking' me on my actual gifts, which was frustrating at the time, but I didn't know why. I put everything down to a lack of intelligence!

The truth is, intelligence is multidimensional. It's not all academic. Imagine a person who is great at creating relationships with people all over the world, but never tried to make it in business because they were rubbish at algebra and failed their maths exams. The world would miss out because it didn't value their emotional intelligence. Now picture somebody who was terrible at running and came last in every race. They might not seem in any way suited to the world of sport when measured by a results-focused model, but what if they could read social situations really well and knew exactly how to encourage others to excel in sport? Those skills are an invaluable asset and could lead to a career in coaching athletes.

Historically, subjects at school didn't reward emotional intelligence or the attuned awareness that some people have, but when robotics are able to replace most jobs, emotional intelligence − this uniquely *human* intelligence − will not fail us.

Going deep

Cultivating emotional intelligence means you become fascinated by emotions, which expands your capacity to go more deeply into them. Wherever I go, people often tell me, "Wow, I don't meet people as deep as you are very often." Here's what I think they're picking up on when they say that. Whenever I enter into a conversation, I love to look at what someone is telling me from about a million different angles as I am fascinated by humans and why we feel the way we do. Often, this looks like asking lots of questions and holding space while they share their truth (more on holding space in a moment). I can sense when someone holds back and will ask appropriate − or sometimes inappropriate! − questions to uncover more and more. I like to go to that depth, which makes the connection between us supercharged. It's all about the depth for me!

As you improve your EQ and start to share how you feel, the emotional depth will come through in your connections and relationships. People will notice. People will start to 'get' you. More like-minded thinkers will become attracted to you.

When I share anything about my life on social media, one of the reasons it is relatable is because I share from an authentic and vulnerable place. I may be sharing something that happened in the past, but I'm not talking about it from a disconnected place. I could say I had a hard time a few years ago, recount what went wrong, and leave it there. But instead, I go more deeply into how it made me feel and what emotion was present. I time-travel back to that place and remember how I sometimes felt really lost, miserable and alone. I recall how I was a little bit happy, but that something made me uncertain and something else made me feel frustrated. When I write that kind of thing, people relate to me and I feel seen. They connect with my humanness because they relate not necessarily to the story but to the feeling.

Sometimes people reject my deepness, saying I'm 'sooooo deep' like it's a bad thing! I have learned to take it as a compliment and simply give them their space. It's okay to operate on a different level from people in your life. Just be you. The most 'you' that you can be. If that's deep, then deep it is. Yey for deep thinkers!

Filling yourself from within

It's all very well to identify emotions in yourself and be able to connect more deeply with yourself and others, but there is one missing piece that we must address when it comes to emotions. What if we can't feel anything? I call this the inner void, and it's that empty hollow pit in your stomach, where you may feel something is lacking or missing, or just not quite right. It is an emotional state of lack, and it's important to mention, because, as we've discussed, we attract more of what we are, so we want to avoid attracting lack or emptiness.

The only way to heal
yourself is to fully

feel your emotions.

You have to go into them
and through them
to reach the other side.

PS I Love Me
www.ginaswire.com

This sense of void is another perception. It is only an issue if you are attached to feeling filled up the whole time. The void is not real. Yes, you may feel it, but at the depths of our being we aren't actually empty, not physically, spiritually or on any level. Although the anatomy of a woman is 'hollow' and a man can 'fill her', perhaps giving her a feeling of 'wholeness', I used to take this too literally, thinking something external was the answer to feeling whole.

Of course, anything external cannot truly fill us because something external can always disappear. When we are only able to be filled by relying on something or someone external to acknowledge us, love us from the outside, it can and will always be taken away. Only when we fill ourselves up from the inside can the fulfilment never be taken away. Filling ourselves with self-love means it's always there, it's endless, it's infinite.

Holding space for yourself is how you ensure you stay filled from the inside. Holding space means everything is allowed, every feeling, every experience. An example of holding space is when I run a retreat and create a container for all the women who attend to feel safe through whatever comes up during our time there. They may experience feelings of pain, sadness, gladness, lack, fear, supercharged joy, terror, anger and everything in between. They may hate what comes up. They may hate me. But any experience arising in the space I welcome and allow, because every emotion is teaching us something.

This is the kind of space you can hold for yourself, space for anything to show up, no matter if it's compassionate or self-loathing. Because, if you're only there for yourself when things are going well, when you're in an emotional state that feels comfortable, you are not really there for yourself at all. That's conditional love, like only loving a child when they're well-behaved. What about the times when there's discomfort? What about the parts that are not pleasant? Can you hold space for that? Because if you can be with the totality of who you are, that is when you are truly flying the self-love flag for all women. You become a walking permission slip for others to rise. And now more than ever, we need YOU, and anyone who is willing, to fly the self-love flag for humanity. So that our children can grow up in a world where self-love is the norm, not the exception.

I often see the ladies who come on my retreats judging themselves or others for their experience if it's not 'positive'. For example, if someone gets triggered and storms out, the other ladies could say, "She shouldn't have done that. It was rude." But actually, this can happen when we stir up old emotions! I just hold space and say, "You focus on you. Send her love and let her have her experience." And this could be a mantra for life! Let everyone have their experience. It's oh-so-freeing!

Staying present

Emotions can hook us and pull us back to our stories. As we know, we all have stories. As humans, we live by stories. We can remember stories from the past and we can also imagine stories for the future.

Truly, though, all we have is now, this present moment. And in the now, stories do not mean anything, nor do they matter. This doesn't mean just forget everything that ever happened to you. However, there is power when you can drop into the now. Something really magical happens when you are able to stay present with yourself and your emotions.

When we identify too rigidly with our story it can keep us stuck. We can't forgive, we can't forget, and we can't move on. When we stop attaching to our stories though, emotional energy can move faster around the body. This is what it means when we say emotions are impermanent. Everything is impermanent, all-flowing, all-moving, all-magical.

Presence is knowing this impermanence, knowing that the void we all feel is not real, and that we can always feel held and safe in a motherly, warm 'womb space'. We can hold the belief that we live a full life from the inside, without being dependent on anything from the outside. Anything that comes in from the outside can be seen as a massive bonus, but it's not sustainable to rely on the outside world to fulfil us. As creators of our whole experience, emotional fulfilment comes from the inside and staying present helps us to remember that we have a choice over how we process our emotions. We can't choose to never feel pain, but we can choose not to suffer.

PS Here's Your Self-Love Medicine

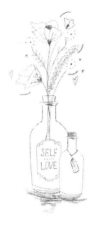

Got some uncomfortable emotions going on? Let's get these emotions out on to paper so you can't hide from them! What emotions are you uncomfortable with?

With your new awareness after this chapter, what three practices are you going to use this week to get more in tune with your emotions and increase your EQ?

CHAPTER SIX

Are You Walking Your Self-Talk?

"Reality is just too real for most of us, so we
temper it with the mind."

Michael A. Singer

Are the thoughts in your head running the show? Is your inner mean girl not shy around a megaphone? Is your mind causing you to doubt yourself with its tricks? These voices that we listen to every day are known as self-talk, and if we don't learn how to interact with them in a mindful way, they can turn into a real drain on our ability to bring good things into our lives and may sabotage the self-love you've already cultivated. Negative self-talk makes you think that your body isn't good enough, it makes you think people don't like you and it makes you stop yourself from doing those scary things (like publishing a book about self-love) in case people don't like it!

I can never
be abandoned again.
I am already chosen,
as I choose myself.
I self-source love
and worthiness
from within.

Love is infinite

In step six of the self-love transformation, you'll learn how to master your self-talk so that you can go ahead and do what you want to do without holding yourself back.

In his book *The Untethered Soul*, Michael Alan Singer describes negative self-talk as like living with an obnoxious roommate and never asking them to leave.

Picture this... You live with housemates who are constantly negative. Just as you're ready to go out, they will point out how terrible you look. They say rude things about how ugly you are, how fat you are, how skinny you are. They remind you that you didn't go to the gym and should have done better. They doubt you too, always questioning the decisions you've made: "Are you really going to launch that project? Are you sure you're ready to ask for a raise?"

Now imagine this... You live in an apartment with some of the most positive people you know, and every day feels like being on holiday with your best friends, who are super supportive and always there for you. When you set out to do something, they tell you that you can do it. You trust that they want the best for you. They tell you how beautiful you are and can always look on the bright side of any situation and see the benefit.

Compare the two. Which set of people would you most like to live with? It's obvious, right? You'd choose to live with the positive ones. Why? Because you can tell that this would have a really positive impact on your life.

The non-judgmental observer

If you want a self-love transformation, becoming conscious of your self-talk will have a huge impact. I say 'becoming conscious' rather than 'shutting down' the negativity, because the aim is to become a non-judgmental observer. Please know that this self-talk is never going away completely. The best we can hope for is to take control of our self-talk, so that we can experience huge leaps forward in life.

The reason that self-talk is not going away is because it has a very important purpose. It is designed to keep us safe. When we are about to do something great, bold or at the edge of our comfort zone, a voice of doubt kicks in. The voice is trying to keep us small because it senses risk and danger. When our ancestors were about to hunt a bear, this was helpful. If the voice said, "That bear's going to kill you", it was our self-talk looking after us, keeping us safe. The problem is, we are not actually in grave physical danger all the time, and self-talk can stop us doing things that may *seem* scary but are actually positive. 'Scary' is subjective and depends on the projection of the mind of each person. Self-talk creates the scariness to keep us safe, but the circumstances themselves may not actually require that protection mechanism.

One day, when I was about to walk on stage at the Bali Spirit Festival – interestingly, to speak about self-talk – it happened to me. I started doubting myself, judging myself and questioning whether the people in the audience were even going to learn anything from me. As I spoke, I started critiquing myself: "You should've done that better. You missed a bit out. What the hell are you on about?" As you see, nobody is exempt from self-talk, but what helped me carry on were the tools I had to deal with it as it happened.

PS I Love Me Practice

One of the tools I love to use is to imagine my thoughts as physical items to 'deal with' another time. Here's how the practice works.

1. Take some deep breaths and start to notice what's in your mind. Observe the thoughts that are coming up. Identify what your doubts are.

2. Now imagine a shelf beside you. Take the thoughts or doubts out of the top of your head and place them on the shelf next to you.

   You can imagine the thoughts or doubts as funny little gremlins laughing at you or taunting you with, "We're your doubts. We're your doubts."

3. Line them up, every single one, and say to them, "I'll deal with you later."

4. If the thoughts or doubts keep going after that, imagine picking up a softball and throwing it at the gremlins lined up on the shelf. Watch them falling onto the floor one by one. It may sound silly, but it deals with the self-doubt in the moment.

5. When you say you'll deal with your gremlins later, the key part is that you *do* come back and face that self-doubt. Take the time to look at each self-doubting thought, acknowledge them one by one, asking yourself this question:

   What is the truth?

No easy bypassing. Take responsibility, work out what those doubts are and meet those fears. Naming them helps you overcome them. If you don't do this, they will keep coming back in to be healed.

Here are some more helpful questions to journal on when examining those gremlins.

How do I deal with this?

How can I choose something else?

Who would I be without that thought?

What's an alternative positive thought?

How would it feel to think that one for a while or forever?

As with blocks and triggers, which we talked about in Chapter Four, self-doubt is all about perception. You can choose what you want to believe. You can choose to believe that you are safe. In the example I gave, this would look like telling myself, "It is safe for me to speak at Bali Spirit Festival. It is safe for me to push the boundaries of my comfort zone. It is safe for me to share my message with the world."

When we speak our *chosen* beliefs out loud, we are programming ourselves to go to the edge of our comfort zone and then beyond it, not just stay home and get smaller. We get to choose – how fun is that?

Finding the intention

Another way you can use self-talk to your advantage is by discovering how those doubts in your mind are trying to help you. Just because self-talk is 'negative' doesn't mean that it is there to be horrible or sinister or prevent you from doing what you want. Remember, self-talk is trying to help you stay safe. Just like in the example of helping you not get killed by a bear, your self-talk might be 'helping you' not rock the boat or 'helping you' not be too awesome so you don't intimidate people you love. It is important to find the intention behind the doubt so that you can make conscious choices.

What negative consequences is your self-talk trying to protect you from? Commonly, self-talk tries to prevent you from creating a situation that you may not want to address right now. Once you look closely at your self-talk to see why it's there, you can choose in your conscious mind whether you do want to address it or not.

Ultimately, all self-talk is self-judgment, so notice the situations that your mind is trying to get you to avoid and see where your comfort zone ends. You can practise this by noticing your friends' and family's self-talk too, although, just as before, keep it to yourself. The purpose of noticing is to help you practise your awareness, not to become the judgmental friend or family member!

Acceptance versus positivity

Although self-talk is trying to help, it is usually ineffective in helping you achieve what you truly want. It drains your energy and causes you to shrink and take up less space. That is the opposite of what you want from life. Self-love is all about opening your heart, taking up *more* space and moving forwards unapologetically. And so, to have a life where you do more of what you love, not less, and become more of who you want to be, not shrink, you'll need to overcome negative self-talk.

As you have already seen earlier in this book, thoughts and stories are just perception, and self-doubt is no different. Doubts are not the truth. However, responding with resistance, such as 'No, none

Our triggers
become our teachers.

of that is true' is not the answer. As we saw earlier, the more you push against something, the more you pull it towards you. Trying to smother the negative self-talk with positive self-talk doesn't work either. Instead, once you identify the doubts, the next stage of overcoming them is to choose to accept exactly *where* you are.

Let's imagine you went to a gym to find a new personal trainer. Maybe you're feeling overweight, you don't feel good in your gym gear, and some of the self-talk that got you here sounded something like, "You need to get yourself to the gym. You're fat. You're overweight. You're gross." Now let's say the gym instructor said those things to you too. "It's a good job you're in the gym. You're fat and disgusting. You should've been here a year ago." Even though you've probably been saying those things to *yourself*, you would probably walk out.

Compare that to a gym instructor who meets you where you are right now. They might speak to you in an encouraging way and say, "Okay, great. You have some goals. You have some weight to lose. You're in the right place. Well done for coming. I'm going to help you. I'm going to show you all the best techniques to help you reach your fitness goals. You haven't done anything wrong. Let's bring you back into harmony." If you were met with acceptance like this, you would stay at the gym, wouldn't you? And you would be more likely to meet your goals.

Note how our imaginary gym instructor was not forcing the *opposite* message. They were not pushing away the negativity with positivity and saying, "You're so beautiful. You're so slim." This is not acceptance, and it wouldn't work because it's not believable. You wouldn't stay at the gym and reach your goals because you wouldn't trust this viewpoint.

Meeting yourself where you are is how you overcome negative self-talk. Not with 'positive' self-talk, but by talking to yourself in a kind, compassionate, encouraging way. Even though a certain amount of self-talk might kick you into touch and motivate you for a while, acceptance is the only way around the confusing push-pull of positive and negative self-talk.

I have experienced the change in my own life. When I was a model, I used to compare myself to others all the time and have a lot of negative self-talk, especially on my way to castings. There would be the negative, "I don't think I've done my makeup well enough." Then the positive, "No, no, no. You're beautiful." Then the negative, "You're probably not going to get the job, because your figure's not good enough." Then the positive, "You're fantastic. You'll nail it. You're going to get the job." By the time I got to the casting, I didn't know where I was or what I thought. I would be all up in my head, feeling like a total mess. A few years on, I have a different approach, just like when stepping on stage at Bali Spirit Festival. I would accept myself where I am and reply to my self-talk, "No, thank you, I don't need to listen to this", and put the doubts on the shelf to deal with later. It's that simple.

It's not a case of having to make the negative positive. All you need to do is choose to accept yourself where you are right now. Even if you have to consciously choose acceptance 1,000 times a day at first, like I did, do it, because it works!

At this point, you may be throwing your book into the sea (here's hoping you are on a lovely beach reading this transmission) or chucking your Kindle out the window. I get it. I've spoken these words many times on retreats and seen bewildered faces staring back at me desperately and passionately wanting to know, "But Gina, *how* do I accept myself? How do I make different choices?"

What I will say here is that if there's one person in the world who is ready to love you, it's you. You have to train yourself to keep coming back to that one true love over and over again. Trust the process, trust the book, trust me. This repeated choosing is the work. Many women who come on a retreat choose to trust, and this is where the magic happens. Possibility expands. Love flows in.

A woman on one of my UK retreats came in seriously lacking any sign of self-love. In fact, she hated herself. She couldn't even bear to look at her own reflection in a mirror. On the second day of the retreat, before our self-love movement practice, she came to me and said, "This morning, I lay in bed listening to the radio and had a sudden urge to hug myself. I heard a voice that just kept saying, *'It's okay, you've been through so much, I'm here for you now, I've been incredibly hard on you and I'm not going to do that anymore.'*" This lady was completely elated as we walked to breakfast together. Grinning and beaming all the way, she kept asking me, "Can it really be that simple? I just have to trust and keep coming back to love?"

The truth is, it's not *easy* but it is *simple*

Self-love is really only ever just one thought away. If you're being hard on yourself, and choosing to love yourself just feels impossible, go back to Chapter One and remind yourself of the cuteness hack. When we notice our cuteness, we acknowledge that our little human doesn't know all the answers yet and that's okay. Cuteness crowds the space where the critic would come in. There's no space for the voices of self-doubt because we reconnect to our humanness and how cute we are, stumbling around trying to figure things out. Becoming hyperaware of your self-talk is a great way to increase your self-love straight away. It's a complete game-changer actually. The kinder and more empathetic you are to yourself, the more you will radiate and flourish in all areas of your life.

PS Here's Your Self-Love Medicine

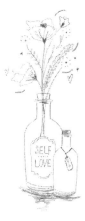 Write a list of all the mean, belittling things you say to yourself regularly. If you are finding it challenging to recount them, think back to the last time you were really upset, triggered or about to do something scary for you. The thoughts should pop up nicely then.

What does your negative self-talk say?

What are these thoughts trying to keep you safe from? What would be a more effective way to speak to yourself?

If you'd like to quieten the voices in your head and love what you see in the mirror, try my *Five-Minute Magic Mirror Boost* at www.ginaswire.com/bookresources.

CHAPTER SEVEN

Comparison, You Are Under Arrest

"Comparison is the thief of joy."

Theodore Roosevelt

Comparison is a big, huge, mahoosive obstruction that prevents us from loving ourselves. If we can eliminate or limit comparison, our self-love will flourish.

As we are heavily influenced by mainstream conditioning, we need to understand why we compare ourselves and how we end up feeling the way we do. In this chapter we will look at why comparison steals away our self-love: how we've fallen for social conditioning; why we can't experience love on the inside while we're comparing ourselves on the outside and how we can stop comparing ourselves so that we can reclaim our self-love.

Exploring your triggers and blocks
increases your self-awareness,
which grows your capacity to love.
The more you know yourself,
the more you can

love yourself.

This is the pathway to
being, getting and having
what you want in your life.

PS I Love Me
www.ginaswire.com

Competition is our conditioning

Social media, advertisements, packaging, TV, film, magazines; what we hear, see, watch and read... Conditioning comes from everywhere. The media industry is built around making us feel like we're not good enough so that we buy or consume what they're selling.

I notice the extent of the media's conditioning whenever I leave Bali and head back to life in the West. One of the joys of living in Bali is that there is so much less consumerism. When I'm in Bali, I'm probably not going to drive past a bus with a giant advert on the side telling me that my teeth aren't white enough. Especially where I live, in Ubud, considerably fewer people watch television, and I don't tend to see magazines with adverts telling me how to fix my cellulite or make my hair shinier.

In the West, we are surrounded by it. Everywhere we go, we receive the message that we need to buy more, more, more. With this kind of marketing all around us, we think we need to *be* more, *do* more, *have* more. It's no wonder we compare ourselves constantly against what everyone else is, does or has.

In a way, Western culture cultivates a sense of lack, distracting us from our emotional pain. Rather than encouraging us to seek solutions within ourselves, we are told to search for quick fixes in the form of the clothes we wear, the things we buy and the type of sex we're having. Consumption and chasing a better version of ourselves is a massive bypass and distraction from the root of it all: the deep fear of not belonging or not feeling loved, AKA all of our emotional baggage. Yet, instead of taking the time to figure out who we are, we spend many years of our lives just trying to fix, fix, fix ourselves. Constantly trying to fit the mould of who we think we should be, who we're being told to be. Being different isn't encouraged. Having an opinion isn't encouraged. We're told we must fit in, not stand out. So, we look around us to see what others are doing and then try to make ourselves more like that. Comparison is a measure of how well we are doing at the task of fitting in.

And it's not just the media telling us to fit in, but the way the whole system is set up, because it's much easier to control people who don't ask too many questions. Desperately trying to fit in also distracts us from asking too many questions of ourselves as well.

Compare and despair

Imagine a scenario where you find yourself comparing your life with someone else's. Usually, you're unaware that you're even doing it. It's passive or mindless. It's not like you put aside dedicated time for it. You don't say to yourself, "Right, now I'm going to sit and compare myself to this woman on Instagram." Usually, it happens when we lose our presence and are not fully in the moment.

Joy, on the other hand, is full presence. Joy is about living fully in the moment. Which means that joy and comparison don't coexist, because comparison means dwelling on the different life choices that we have made to get to where we are. Knowing this can be helpful if you catch yourself on Instagram looking at all your friends who are married with babies, while you are single, or find yourself thinking about wealthy friends who chose a corporate career path, while you live out of a backpack. As always, we come back to the act of making a conscious choice.

During my modelling years, I had a habit of going on to my agency website and clicking through every single picture of the other models on there. Guess how much negative self-talk that would spark?! I would flick through the photos comparing myself: "Her career is better than mine. She's more toned than I am. She's smoother than I am. She's taller than I am." I would kid myself that it was constructive criticism, but here's the problem with that. For some of us, criticism can't be constructive because it makes us far less likely to want to do something. It can make us want to shrink rather than grow.

So just as joy and comparison can't sit in the same container, nor can we pretend that comparison is a method of constructive criticism.

What you miss when you're in your head

It's not about setting out to feel bad. It's not that you're trying to punish yourself deliberately. It's not that you think you'll make yourself feel better by being mean. It's a conditioned response. We think, "Oh, she looks nice." Then that thought pattern soon turns into, "Oh, she's nicer than me, so that means I'm not going to be loved."

Comparison becomes a problem when we believe another person's beauty, success or worth could jeopardise the love we'll receive or the opportunities we will be given. Comparison can be natural and healthy if we are able to appreciate and be inspired by the beauty, success or worth of another person. Notice how that is a completely different energy to the negative feeling of competing for love and opportunities. Feeling under threat is not conducive to helping you to expand and improve, and it prevents you from being who you truly are. It can even make you miss out on the joy you have right in front of you.

This happened to Paige, a member of my Infinite Self-Love Society Facebook group, a free group for women who want to drop the self-doubt and embrace themselves more fully. Paige posted about her experience of comparison and the downward spiral of self-loathing that she experienced by not being present in the moment. She talked about how she went to a concert with her partner and spent the whole night thinking she wasn't as pretty as the other women, not as skinny as them, not as cool as them, not as successful as them, not as tall as them, not as fashionable as them... Paige was so in her head, comparing herself to other women, feeling worthless, giving herself a hard time and even imagining her partner of three years leaving her for one of these women, that she didn't even remember seeing Drake, the artist she had so madly wanted to see.

I can relate! When I was younger, I would spend three hours getting ready for a night out with my friends, trying to make myself look perfect. I would scrutinise myself in the mirror thinking my tan should be darker, my lashes longer, and that I definitely should have figured out a regular gym routine by this stage in my life. After a lot of vodka, I wouldn't care so much and I'd feel ready to leave the house. Some nights out I'd be absolutely fine; confident, enjoying myself and being social. Often, these were the nights where I was getting a lot of male attention from the get-go. Then I would ride that wave of attention to feel good (hello outside validation!). It's embarrassing to say this now, but honestly, I would think that these 'good' nights were down to the dress I was wearing or how well I'd done my makeup. That dress would go into the 'wear again' section of my wardrobe!

Other nights I would feel like I was invisible and go into complete comparison mode. I'd see a perfectly toned women in a perfectly fitting designer dress getting chatted up by a man I fancied, and it was game over. In this headspace, fun went out the window and the whole night was spent in my head wishing I could look better and be more attractive. Needless to say, that dress would be in the charity shop pile and never worn again. Ever! That's how it worked.

The sad part of this is that those women I perceived to be so beautiful or popular or together or successful or wealthy may have been comparing themselves to other women in the wine bar too.

If you can be with the totality of who you are, that is when you are truly flying the

self-love flag

for all women.

PS I Love Me
www.ginaswire.com

Perhaps they had their own internal emotional struggles or their own hang-ups about how they looked or came across. A friend of mine, Rianne, summed this up perfectly in my Infinite Self-Love Society Facebook group (come join us!). She said that she stopped comparing herself to others the day the woman she'd compared herself to for years, told her that she'd always compared herself to Rianne!

The difficulty with comparison is that it isn't an accurate measure of where we are at all. Everything is down to perception. I may have a perception that a particular woman is the most beautiful, eye-catching woman in the room, but that doesn't necessarily mean she loves herself or is more desirable. The woman who has great energy about her will be the one who is truly radiant. The woman who feels great in her body becomes a magnet to whatever she wants. It's about how you show up, how you feel, how your confidence comes through and how much fun you're having, not having the smoothest thighs or the most symmetrical face. It's your energy. It doesn't matter what your perception or judgment of everyone else is. It only matters how you perceive and judge yourself.

Comparison is all in the head, so we've got to get out of the head if we're going to solve the comparison problem. The great news is that knowing it's a perception means we can choose a different perception. Let's go back to the wine bar and imagine what I might say to myself instead of staying in comparison mode. If I was present enough to catch myself comparing, I could remind myself that comparison and joy can never live in the same container and ask... *What could I choose instead?*

Better choices

When comparison becomes a problem and you perceive that others have something you don't, it is a barrier to attracting what you want. When a woman is empowered and has self-love, she becomes a magnet to everything she desires. When a woman desperately lacks confidence and visibly struggles to accept herself, that struggle is what is felt around her. That energy perpetuates. That is why it's so important to choose joy over comparison. It will ripple through the rest of your life and what you manifest.

Now you know this, it is up to you to make a different choice.

PS I Love Me Practice

Choosing joy will cultivate self-love. Here are some ideas to play with that will lessen comparison and expand self-love. I invite you to choose one and commit to doing it this week:

- Put on a happy playlist and dance like everybody is watching! Or nobody! Whatever makes you feel good! Whack on my *Infinite Self-Love Playlist* – www.ginaswire. com/bookresources – if you need some help getting in the zone and unleashing your inner wild woman.

- Go to the mirror and speak your gratitude practice out loud. Include yourself, your body and each and every part of you for everything she does for you each day.

- Find a comfortable place to soak up some positive conditioning. Read a book that makes your heart sing or listen to an inspiring podcast.

- Call a good friend who gets it. Admit what you've been thinking, even if you are in tears as you do, then laugh about how tragic yet cute we humans are. We're all a bit lost at times, and laughter helps us move through it. *Best friends, I salute you. You know who you are. Thank you.*

- If you don't have women in your life who you can turn to like this, feel free to join the Infinite Self-Love Society Facebook group. This is where the cool open women hang out, share and support each other!

- Cuddle a puppy or visualise cuddling one. *This one works well for me!*

When you first start doing this, you might have to choose joy over comparison 1,000 times a day. That was certainly my experience. If I felt tempted to compare myself to other models on the agency website or if I was going into an Instagram hole, I would have to switch off my laptop. Put away my phone. Shut off. Choose joy. Go and do something else.

Comparison becomes irrelevant

There's another choice to make too, and that is the choice to know you are worth it and see your own beauty. There is beauty in everyone, and finding your gift will be invaluable. Whether that's showing up as the kindest person, being loving, having a message to share or exuding energy that makes people feel happy and free, you can accentuate that aspect of yourself. Tune in and grow from that place and your beauty will be seen. That's what it means to be truly beautiful from the inside, to know your gifts and how to use them. People think that it's wrong to 'feed the ego' but owning your gifts can be both humble and generous. It's not about trying to be something you're not. It's knowing on a soul level that we're all made of the same stuff. We are all born worthy and there is space for everybody.

It's natural to see what other people are doing and want a piece of that for yourself, but only by having your own vision and becoming more of your own essence will you become a magnet to opportunities. It never works when people copy others or try to emulate people who are doing fantastically well. If you can stand in your own essence with your own vision, even in a saturated space, you can do well for yourself.

If you need an example of this, look at the thousands of self-love and transformation coaches out there. It would be easy to think there wasn't space for one more, but I looked at it differently. A huge vision is guiding me. I want to help a billion women overcome their inner struggles so they can live with purpose and passion. When I tune in to that vision, there is no competition. When I teach from my story, from my heart, from my experience, there is no competition. Everyone's essence is unique and nobody else has your story.

Imagine you want to become a coach or yoga teacher or leader of some kind. If you sit on the sidelines watching the big players, it's easy to think you could never do what they do, or criticise those who are in the game when they get something wrong. However, let's look at it like this. Those people who are in the game, showing up every day, putting themselves out there, taking risks and throwing themselves out of their comfort zone to receive opportunities and greatness, they don't criticise the people on the sidelines. They're in the game. It's difficult to be happy as a spectator, because spectators are constantly comparing themselves. Once you're in the arena, it doesn't matter if you win or lose, because there are no failures, only lessons.

When you know who you are and connect with your vision, comparison isn't even an option. At the start, you will need to choose and choose and choose joy over comparison every time. Eventually, though, once you truly step into the arena and transform, removing your blocks and stepping into your power, you won't need to make that choice as often. Comparison will dissipate until it is no longer much of a consideration at all because you are *there* and you're *doing it.*

When I stepped into the arena myself, this is exactly how it happened for me. Even though I was good at it, modelling was never really a passion for me, so when I quit and took charge of my life, I became more aligned. I started saying yes to everything that was a true yes and no to everything that was just a maybe or a full no. Doing this allowed that huge vision to come through, which meant there was much less space for comparison. It just didn't enter my head anymore.

Comparison stops being a problem when you are in your essence, striving towards your vision, guided by your passion and purpose. If you are at the beginning of your journey with comparison, first choose joy, but also know that there is more for you out there. As you grow your awareness and let your essence naturally unfold, you will reach the point where you skyrocket into empowerment and self-love. And comparison melts away.

The truth of our being is that we don't need to walk around telling everyone about how powerful we are. We don't need to out-twerk our best mate to prove that we are powerful. We don't need to try to be the most magnetic woman in the room. We don't need to have the best-dressed pooch, the swankiest wheels, the deepest tan, the longest lashes or the trendiest bum shape of the century. The truth of our being just quietly *knows* and therefore *chooses* not to have to prove anything to anyone. It resides in the clear, quiet, grounded place of understanding self.

We are mahooosively disconnected as a society. We run around like headless chickens trying to get love or trying to be someone different so we can get love, but reconnection with our personal power means that we no longer need to look to our parent, our peer group or Peter-with-the-eight-pack who we met that one time in the club, because we damn sure know who we are. That is where your power comes from. And that reconnection to self is always just one thought away.

PS Here's Your Self-Love Medicine

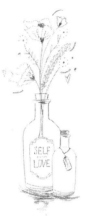

Isn't it time to quit the comparison? Reflect on times when comparison has stolen your self- love.

It's time to celebrate your uniqueness. Write a list of everything that makes you uniquely you, including quirks, beauty, personality, friends, talents, lifestyle and anything else that is special about you. Aim for 50 items. (Minimum 20!)

CHAPTER EIGHT

Just a Soul Having a Human Experience

"and i said to my body. softly. 'i want to be your friend.' it took a long breath. and replied 'i have been waiting my whole life for this.'"

Nayyirah Waheed

Self-love is being, doing and having more of the things you love in your life, and this includes loving the 'bad' bits, the wobbly bits, the aspects of our beings we'd rather nobody knew about, the dark and glorious desires that reside within. Simply put, it's about embracing the whole blessed thing! Nothing is exempt. Everything is welcome.

Living in the body we were given can be a challenge for many of us. So much so that the term 'body acceptance' has come into existence. In step eight, you will learn how to find a new appreciation for your body by tuning into the frequency of gratitude and expansion,

＊＊＊ ❤ ＊＊＊

If there's one person
in the world who is ready
to love you, *it's you!*
You have to train yourself to keep
coming back to that one true love
over and over again.

PS I Love Me
www.ginaswire.com

getting to the truth of the matter when it comes to caring for your body, rather than abandoning yourself.

What does it look like when we abandon ourselves? This could be any way of acting that is not self-loving. For example, hating yourself because you ate something you don't normally eat, deciding you've screwed up so you might as well eat the cake, binge-drink or go all out in some way, shutting the door in your own face, not being a friend to yourself, telling yourself you should know better or that you're an idiot.

For me, my self-abandonment was always around eating. I would be in a super healthy state of going to spin class and hot yoga or hanging by my knees from straps doing push-ups against the gym wall, then, after a wholesome raw vegan organic superfood salad wrapped in a giant kale leaf with my yoga buddies, I'd end up frantically eating a four-pack of giant New York triple chocolate muffins on the way home. I would yo-yo between those two states, but I really knew I'd abandoned myself when my thoughts turned nasty. "What an idiot, you've just worked out and then ruined it all, what's the actual point?! Useless. You can't stick to anything. That's it. From tomorrow, the only thing you're allowed is green juice." And this soulless cycle would repeat. Gym, eat, berate, repeat.

You were fine all the time

I used to reject parts of my body: the shape of my breasts; the ripples of cellulite; the look of my feet. I used to particularly dislike my toes and would plan a whole outfit around making sure no one would see my feet. I always wore socks and would never go barefoot, which is crazy to imagine now.

It's not that I followed a formula to help me love my body. As far as I know, there wasn't one at that time anyway. Like I've mentioned before, I didn't have a guide or mentor to support me with this.

Based on what I've learned and what has worked for my clients, I have now created this step-by-step process to help speed things up for you. Yey!

At a certain stage of your self-love transformation, you will realise (as I realised) that there isn't any need to change anything about your body! At first, this was a strange feeling, as someone who had been completely consumed with bettering my body for years. It wasn't that I *tried* to accept my body and suddenly it had worked. It was that I no longer *needed* to accept myself. It was already done. It was like I had remembered that I was fine all along.

Although I had spent a long time rejecting myself, my body was always still there, always doing its job. Your body is your home, so wherever you are in the world, you are already home.

Like I explained in the previous chapter, a lot of our critical self-talk isn't there because there is something inherently wrong with us, but because of how we are conditioned to think about ourselves. When we were small children, we didn't think, *OMG my arms are too fat* or, *Yikes! My feet are the wrong size.* We never focused on changing our hair colour (unless we got to have one of those epic hair braids with a jewel on the end, which I begged my parents for every time we went on holiday for years. I was finally allowed one and got to keep it in for school! Winning!).

As we grow up, the more we forget who we truly are – a soul having a human experience – the more we get caught up in what our bodies 'should' look like. Shifting our acceptance starts with the remembrance of ourselves as souls rather than humans. It can be so inspiring to broaden the perception outside the physical body.

I should note here that, when I had this realisation, it wasn't like I was suddenly ecstatic about my body. I felt neutral. There was no negativity, but no positivity either. It just was what it was.

And if anybody didn't like my body, that was fine too. I was no longer interested in other people's opinions of my body, because I accepted myself.

Is it time for you to remember that you have been fine this whole time?

A new appreciation

Not only are our bodies just fine as they are, but they do so much for us. Reminding ourselves of everything our bodies do gives us a new appreciation for them. The shift from *having* to accept your body to the idea of *remembering* who you are makes so much sense when you think about how incredible human beings are. Our brain works non-stop. Our digestion works non-stop. Our body is in a constant state of cleansing. It is fascinating and fantastic.

Yet it is not unusual to forget our amazingness. We humans have a frequent state of amnesia around this miracle. We tend to forget that our bodies are all good. They are doing a job. They don't need to change what they are doing, and they don't need us constantly trying to change them.

Realising this can show us where we have been unfair on our bodies, which are constantly supporting us, and yet often we don't love them in return. Imagine you were in a relationship with someone who never showed up for you and wasn't loving or supportive, while you were giving it your all and being super kind all the time. It's likely you would end up resenting the other person. Your body is no different. If your body is always showing up for you, but if you're always mean to it, it will start to resent you, which means you can manifest problems. Low energy vibes turn into problems, problems into struggles, and struggles into physical manifestations like disease.

So many women who I coach are addicted to stress, which is often a sign that they don't love themselves. I'm not talking about short-term stress when something crazy is happening in your life like a big event or working long days to hit a deadline. I'm talking about the constant stressors that a lot of people carry around with them for long periods of time.

A client of mine, Cath, shared with me that she always has to have her house immaculate in case her in-laws drop by and that she can never stay in her dressing gown past 7am in case someone thinks she is lazy. Underneath all of this was a lack of worthiness, a feeling of inadequacy and that being herself was somehow 'wrong'. Once we dived into this in coaching, Cath realised that she longed to be loved by everybody. So, she put all this extra stress on herself every day. The question is always: *at what cost?*

I've witnessed personally how stress can destroy not just self-love but also life. My dad's early death was a product of stress. I used to wonder why he died of such an aggressive type of oesophagus cancer at 55 when he was super active and fit, ate healthily, drank alcohol infrequently and didn't smoke. I even took the nutrition course in New York because I had this constant thought running through my mind that I couldn't let anybody else around me die of this terrible disease. I knew the food-health connection was important, then I had a huge breakthrough around self-love, which plays a massive part in the amount of stress people carry which hugely affects the physical body.

What I found out about stress was shocking but made sense. Continuous stress (a product of not accepting yourself as you are) raises the heart rate and elevates the levels of stress hormones. This takes its toll on the physical body.

Dad was a busy entrepreneur, active in charity and community work, with two families to look after. I believe he was avoiding a lot of unresolved issues and using 'busyness' to do so. When I started exploring stress, I realised that he may never have truly found what he was looking for in life; he was looking for love and acceptance in all the wrong places. What he truly needed was self-love and self-acceptance.

A holistic way of looking at disease in the body is that it can start in the mind with the way we think about ourselves. It's super important to go into this work by clearing what does not serve us. When we flip the script on our body and the way we feel about it, we change everything. Not just feeling comfortable to wear a cute outfit or showing up confidently, but switching into a full state of gratitude and genuinely appreciating everything your amazing body does for you.

Your body is constantly supporting you in everything you do, which is a complete and utter miracle. We forget that we are a work of art, a soul within a body. If you've ever seen a dead body, you'll understand what I mean, because there is nothing there once the soul has left this physical human plane. We are a combination of solid mass and spirit. Nobody really knows how the soul gets there, but when a baby is born, it's the ultimate miracle.

When you reject any part of yourself or your body – a wonky nose, jibbly thighs, a saggy midriff – it is a very human experience, but also a complete waste. It's time to stick a stake in the ground and powerfully claim the reality that you choose to live in. A reality aligned with how you wish to feel in your skin suit. As you go on this journey of reclaiming your body, know that you are a walking miracle. Your body is an 'exquisite pharmacy' as Deepak Chopra calls it, constantly creating cures for ailments you're not even aware of, because your body's got your back. Literally. When you enter into full gratitude mode for your body, you'll instinctively treat her better. You'll be boosted with happy hormones, and feeling good about yourself will be your natural state.

People respond to this altered energy, and not just because you might dress differently. You could be wearing your gym kit, with slicked back hair, covered in sweat, but if you feel great, you'll have a spring in your step and people will see and feel that. When your energy is higher it lifts those around you. The shell doesn't matter. It's truly about the energy you exude. Equally, you could spend three hours getting ready to go out and wear the most expensive designer outfit, but if you're in a weird mood, feeling unaccepting of yourself and like you're not good enough, the lack of confidence will show. That's what people pick up on.

I'm not saying that you need to force yourself to be high-vibe if you're having one of those days. We are cyclical, seasonal beings. We are supposed to experience all the feelings. Just like when it goes dark at night. We don't sit there and wish it was daylight. We accept the darkness, knowing it will be light again in the morning. Self-love is loving it all. And when you have lower-energy days, like the seasons, know that it will change. And give yourself extra love in the meantime. Like a fire on a cold winter's day, give yourself that extra cosy warmth to get yourself through to the next spring, in your step.

Body BS

When we're in a place of non-acceptance around our body, we might also accept some of the crap stories that other people have about their bodies and the messages they give us. What people say, especially when we are younger, can be so damaging and ultimately untrue. Their motivation can come from a place of being hurt themselves.

When we believe comments or criticisms from the past, they can play out in the life we live today. All through my modelling career I carried the belief that I had fat arms, which I had picked up from someone else's hang up. Remember, this is your life, you only get one body, and YOU get to choose exactly what you believe about her. If you're buying into any outdated, boring AF, low-vibe, mean girl BS that was never yours to begin with, put your hand on your heart, feel your divinity, know that I'm energetically supporting you in your journey and if I can do it, and thousands of other women can do it, you can too. Preach!

You will fluctuate

It's normal to repeat old patterns sometimes, because we move in and out of alignment. And we are supposed to. This journey is not linear. However, after doing some of this self-love work, you might notice that when you do return to old patterns, the period of time getting back to yourself is much shorter. Part of why you are experiencing these repeated lessons is to show you how much you've grown. Yes, you slip, but then life goes on.

Every time I visit England and stay with my mum, I find myself slipping into past habits in that environment. I might go into the fridge in the middle of the night or find myself extra hungry when I'm there, partly because that's how I felt and behaved when I used to live there, and partly because I know my mum always has all the yummy foods that I love and grew up eating. She looks after me so well!

Know that your body, your dedication and your feelings will all fluctuate and that's okay. The key is not to abandon yourself. I've already talked about what abandoning yourself looks like, but here's the thing. It's not actually about the action. If you slip, that's normal, but it's why you slip that you need to look at, because the same action could be motivated by two entirely different feelings. It's about how we *feel* when doing that action.

Let me show you what I mean with an example. I could eat chocolate cake and it be an act of self-love. Let's say I'm out with friends and consciously choosing the chocolate cake, enjoying each mouthful, seeing it as a gift and feeling nourished. Can you see how that's different from eating the cake in a triggered state of feeling like I'm not enough or as a kind of punishment towards myself and the body that makes me feel awful feelings?

We all recognise this downward spiral of beating ourselves up, but you can't hate yourself into a better-feeling body. Feeling good about yourself cannot happen in that space. Only by loving yourself, trusting yourself and appreciating that you can't be optimal all the time, will you bounce back. Tough times happen, going off-piste happens. We all fall into old patterns and lose awareness for chunks of time. But it will start to happen less and less often.

When I was modelling, I would emotional-eat in my hotel rooms or in my car, which looked like eating anything and everything in sight, even if it wasn't that nice. It was about putting it into my body in a desperate kind of way. The best way to explain it is being 'out of my mind', almost like something had taken over me. After it passed, I would call my mum and say, "The monster got me again". It's weird to look back and remember myself doing that. The whole time I needed exactly what this book teaches. In some ways, I'm writing it for the me I used to be back then!

What I'm saying is that it's okay. It's life. We're human! It's about what we learn from these low points and how we use that wisdom to move forward. Your natural state is self-love and harmony, so you can allow yourself to fluctuate without exaggerating the downturns and making more of them than they need to be.

PS I Love Me Practice

If you're going through a tough time, please know that *what you resist will persist!* Find some time to be silent and still. Feel what is truly going on for you, hold space for yourself, give yourself a break, remember it all starts with you. External validation or stuffing yourself with carbs will only soothe you so much. Only self-love will lead you to the satisfaction and harmony you truly crave. I can 100% vouch for this.

In this self-love visualisation, you're going to imagine what it would feel like to love the skin you're in.

1. Take a few moments now to ask yourself this question and visualise the answer.

   If I loved my body fully, how would I show up?

   Close your eyes and imagine how you would walk into a room, how your energy would come over to other people. Would it be confident, sensual, attractive, healthy, happy? If you loved your body fully, how would you show up in the world differently at work, with your partner, in your life and with yourself?

2. Next ask yourself this:

   When you think of loving your body fully, what are you resisting feeling?

   Remember, it's all welcome. Give yourself permission to be less than perfect and love yourself through it. When you don't resist those feelings, you will come back into harmony more quickly.

3. Slowly open your eyes and come back to the book. If you want to pause here and write anything down, feel free.

Body harmony

I know, really well, what disharmony feels like. As I mentioned before, I used to spend two to three hours getting ready for a night out with friends. I'd wear fake tan and fake lashes, and have my nails done with gel. I'd spend many hours and even more money shopping for the perfect backless, frontless, eye-catching, tight, flattering, boob-enhancing, bum-minimising dress, always with new matching everything! Hair had to be perfect. Makeup flawless. All of it had to be 'just so'.

Usually, I would do this stressful ritual with all my friends at my house. Exciting! Or was it? We would drink while we were getting ready. And at every stage, I would outsource my power, my intuition and my likes and dislikes to my friends by constantly asking them what they thought. Sound familiar?

By the time we were ready to go, there would be a photoshoot and lots of self-critiquing. The negative self-talk would be on overdrive, but suppressed and numbed by the alcohol. Wow! Recounting this is fun but also sad.

Once we got to where we were going, I'd be hit or miss. Sometimes, I'd be like a magnet and everybody wanted to talk to me. Other times, it was like I was invisible. Did I have fun standing in a crowded room with super loud music and drunk people that I didn't know rating me on how I looked? Was it enjoyable wearing high heels and tight clothing, wondering if I was good enough and letting strangers decide that for me? Waaaaah! No!

The truth is
it's not *easy*,
but it is *simple*.
Self-love is really
only ever just
one thought away.

Let's compare that to how I get ready now. It looks a lot different and feels a lot more harmonious. Unless I'm doing a self-love ritual, purely to pamper myself, I spend about 10 minutes getting ready. For 90% of the time, I wear my hair in natural waves, makeup minimal, clothing comfy and relaxed. I choose it based on whatever I'm attracted to at the time and what feels fun, joyful and enjoyable to wear. I see myself as a work of art in the mirror and most of the time my inner voice is that of a best friend. My skin beams. My eyes are clear and bright. I enjoy being in my body and I know that she fluctuates. And that's all perfectly in flow.

If I'm not feeling 100%, I reassure my body that she's doing a fabulous job. That she's kind, healthy, helpful, loved, trusted, wanted and free. I choose how I want to feel when I enter a room, and usually have a word or phrase to keep me centred like 'grace' or 'trust' or 'worthy with nothing'.

Yikes! That contrast alone is worth celebrating, and it's totally possible for you too. If you are not at the point yet where you feel you can love and accept yourself as you are, I invite you to show up anyway and keep showing up, because every single time you choose yourself and choose your body, you are showing up for you. It is only a matter of time before you reach that tipping point where everything changes. Choose body-loving, choose to feel amazing about everything your body does for you, every single day.

An especially powerful tip to help you choose body-loving comes from a breakthrough that an amazing lady, Josie, had on one of my retreats. In our famous body acceptance workshops, she suddenly said, "Hold on a minute. I'm too fat for who?"

She was a happily married woman with two gorgeous sons, and yet she had been holding onto the story that she was too fat to receive love for a long time. In actual fact, nobody else was thinking that other than herself. She made the connection that if she decided she wasn't too fat, then nobody thought it anymore. And even if they did, it wasn't a problem for her.

Since then, we've spoken about the massive shift that everyone had that day in that workshop. She's shared how the inner shift she experienced has been reflected across her entire life. Her business is doing better than ever, her negative self-talk has gone away, she's been earning more money, she moved to a lovely big, new house and her relationship with her partner is more joyful than ever.

PS Here's Your Self-Love Medicine

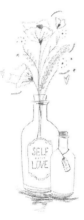

You have the power to think what you want about yourself. This is the magic!

Insert your struggle and reflect on whether it's true:

I'm too _____ for who?

Let that land for a second. If you go deep, the answer always comes back to you. And if it's just you who you need to convince of your worthiness, you have the power.

Which part of your body or face do you usually criticise the most? What's your earliest memory of not loving that part of yourself?

Example: I criticise my thighs because I remember being teased at school by the boys saying I have thunder thighs.

What loving things would you like to tell the younger you who rejected that part of yourself?

Example: Sweetheart, your thighs are perfect as they are. The boys are just being silly. They're children battling the pressures of trying to fit in. It's not the truth. You are loved and lovely just as you are.

CHAPTER NINE

The Power of Choice

"Whatever you are not changing,
you are choosing."

Laurie Buchanan

You choose nearly everything in your world. And yet, there are likely to be things in your life right now that you don't want. The people you allow into your life, the job you do, the passions you have, the partner you decide to stay with – these are all choices. If you haven't actively selected these, then you've *allowed* them into your field.

Equally, you can let go of almost all of it. You are the creator. You are the creative force. You can create whatever you want. Women are capable of creating life itself, the ultimate miracle. If we can create consciousness within our body, we can sure as heaven create a business or a book or a relationship.

Choice is a superpower inside every single person. If we forget this and think we have no choice, we become disempowered. As the

The kinder and more
empathetic you are
to yourself,
the more you will
radiate
and flourish in all
areas of your life.

PS I Love Me
www.ginaswire.com

creator of your life, you really do have to be clear on your vision and make that shit happen!

A series of poor choices gets you into a mess, into blocked, lost, stuck, small, stifled states. And a series of choices gets you out. You can choose anything you want. What do you choose?

Loving yourself is a choice. Choice is a big theme that runs through every chapter of *PS I Love Me*. Take self-talk as an example. What you choose to say to yourself is a choice. With body acceptance, what you choose to think when you look at yourself is a choice. Not comparing yourself to other women or to your old self is a choice. Can you see how important your choices are and that you are the one making them? You are the one with the power to choose whatever you want.

Now it is time to take radical responsibility for all your choices. This is the ninth step of self- love transformation. We make hundreds of choices each day, thousands per month, millions over a lifetime. All these micro-choices add up. The choices you have made in your life so far have led you to where you are right now. You are an amalgamation of all the choices you have made in the past. And you have choice over where you want to go in the future. So, let's dive in.

It starts with intuition

In order to fully love ourselves, we need to start making the most self-loving choices. How do you know which choices are going to be self-loving or not? Intuition helps to guide us towards what will serve us best.

In our modern-day society, gut feelings are often brushed off as 'nothing', yet the gut is starting to be referred to as the 'second brain' because it contains around 100 million neurons. Tuning into the wisdom of the gut is incredibly helpful. The more we listen to this voice, the more we will hear.

We've already talked about trust and intuition in Chapter Three, but to recap, intuition isn't necessarily logic; it may not make sense to you, it's a feeling or hunch, as opposed to what your mind thinks is reasonable. Trusting it can take you into some fantastic spaces within yourself and within the world. It can end up connecting you with the most incredible people and opportunities in the most random places, just because you followed your soul's voice. The other day I was driving through a small town in Bali where you definitely would *not* usually go to buy a dress for a wedding, and I suddenly got an 'intuitive hit' to go into a shop which had all these naff dresses in the window. I went in gingerly and the whole shop was full of frocks that were a full body '*No!*' But there was a tiny section at the back with ten dresses that were all gorgeous and I could have worn any of them; I had the pick of the bunch! Thank you, Universe! More please!

Not where you want to be

Back when I was modelling, even though it *seemed* like a 'dream life', it was not where I wanted to be. It wasn't right for me. It wasn't home for me. I felt out of alignment with myself and didn't know what I wanted. In a word, I was lost.

Have you ever felt lost like that? If so, know that your choices have led you there and your choices can lead you out. Your choices are always right on some level; they may help you to grow, to learn what you *don't* want and lead you to figure out where you need to go next.

At 17, I had gone into modelling for a bit of fun, but I wasn't particularly into fashion and it wasn't something I was desperate to do as a career. My dad and grandparents encouraged me because I got scouted and they were proud. Their encouragement came from a loving place. My mum said I should do it if I wanted to, and my friends said I should definitely go for it. Choosing this path helped to lead me where I needed to go. It served me really well and gave me lots of friends and contacts.

However, towards the end of my modelling career, I wasn't choosing myself, nourishing myself, or following a path that made me alive. I was so far off my centre. The choices I was making didn't fuel my passion. Being in that weird place, I didn't even know that I wasn't choosing myself, let alone understand how I might start. But I did begin to realise that I had been conditioned by forces outside me. At the height of my modelling career, people would ask me, "Where are you going next? When are you going to be in LA? When are you going to be in Paris? When are you going to be in Barcelona?" Inside, I thought that I needed to go to all these places so that people would see me there and I would feel like a success. But by whose definition of success? I needed to discover my own definition of success, from within.

When I left that industry, I reclaimed myself, and started to listen in and ask myself what it would look like if I chose myself and created my own version of success. For me, this looked like quitting modelling at the peak of my career, leaving behind all the fancy clothes and the lifestyle, and following my intuition towards a healthier lifestyle.

Perhaps you recognise this trap of people-pleasing and ego-pleasing, thinking you have to show up as a certain person. Yet only when you drop the facade can you really find yourself. Where in your life do you feel like you're not choosing you? Where does it feel like you're pleasing others by showing up a certain way?

Guided choices

I chose to start following my intuition because this word 'intuition' had come into my field. I started hearing it everywhere. I researched it and learned more and more. I realised that intuition had always been inside me, but I hadn't had the language for it. From the most unaligned place in my life, I started to make some really good choices for myself. At the time, I didn't even know how great they would turn out to be, but a higher force was guiding me. And for the first time in a long time, I was listening. One good choice led to another and another and another…

When I moved from London to New York, I only had one friend, and I recognised that I needed to get creative to meet more people. I made the choice to join a dating app and went out with lots of men because I wanted to make friends and connect with people. Sometimes I was going on dates that I didn't really want to go on, but I went because I was seeking connection.

Suddenly, I was really drawn to practising yoga again. I had done some in the past and had this gut feel to start going again. I did a few classes and liked it, so I bought an unlimited pass. I began going all the time and meeting people who were interested in being healthy, who ate food that was good for them, who talked about wellness topics and had a non-judgmental community where they shared the yoga philosophies.

One teacher was so influential for me and taught a class that blew my mind. What she said and the way she showed up was so radiant. I was used to being surrounded by jaw-droppingly beautiful people in the industry I worked in, and I noticed how she didn't look like them, but had this radiance pouring out of her. She was magnetic, mesmerising, like beaming sunlight. It was the wake-up call I needed to see the difference between models who looked super amazing but had low energy, and a radiant yoga teacher with sky-high energy.

When I heard she was running a course, I signed up immediately. I didn't even know what this 'intuition' thing was all about, but I knew that I wanted to do her course. That course led me to the intuitive nutrition course, which turned out to be the instigator of my self-love career. Almost by accident, I learned how to be a coach, when I thought I was signing up to learn about nutrition.

All of these choices were guided, but as you can see, I could never have understood at the time just how guided, impactful and insightful they would turn out to be. Guided choices might feel at the time that you just want 'a piece of whatever she's having'. You may not know what it is yet, but you know it lights you up. Little by little, as you spend more and more time following the threads of what piques your interest and learning from inspired people, you may make small yet very different choices in your life. And then, you might make a huge leap.

When you make that choice, you may have to hold strong to what you have chosen, as people around you might not always agree with what you're doing, but it's your choice. If you listen to what your gut feeling is telling you to do, you will make better choices for you.

When I started following my inner guidance and making choices based around self-love, people thought I was absolutely bonkers, especially after building my modelling career for so many years to pursue something like yoga that had no guarantees. Here's what I say to that... People *still* think I'm bonkers for the choices I make! Even though I've been living in Bali, working online and travelling the world, I still encounter people who think I made the wrong choice. People will always think you're bonkers when you don't do things the way they do. People say I'm bonkers for continent hopping, doing a 20-day juice fast in the jungle in Costa Rica, spending my time and money trekking to random energy vortexes, sitting with my distance healer over Zoom or chanting into the Ganges sitting next to a couple of cows, rather than rooting in one place, and settling down in a more traditional situ. But that's self-love, people! Making choices with guidance from the inside, not the outside.

The point is, some people choose to do things a certain way, but when I tune in to what my intuition is telling me, what's truly guiding me, this is it. This is the only way it can be for me right now and I trust completely that it will all work out.

When you start to reclaim yourself, listen to yourself and make choices based on your intuition, people might question that. You may even doubt yourself sometimes. You might wonder, "What if they're right?" If that happens, you just need to come back into full trust, knowing that you have your own inner guidance. You are a miraculous being with all these opportunities and all these choices. Trust yourself to make empowered choices, because these choices are guided (and if you struggle with trust, go back and read the trust chapter of this book again!).

Just because your choices are guided doesn't mean that everything will turn out the way you want it to every single time. When something doesn't go the way you hoped, after following your gut, that doesn't mean you can't trust it. You can trust yourself and still end up in a duff situation. If something goes differently to what you'd expected, know that you likely learned something you needed to learn along the way. Or maybe you got to see exactly what you *don't* want in your life, which ultimately clarifies what you do want and leads you towards enlightenment! And that, ladies, is the great paradox of life.

As you grow your awareness
and let your essence naturally
unfold, you will reach the point
where you *skyrocket*
into empowerment
and self-love.

And comparison melts away.

In a way, it means there are no bad choices. Everything that's happening is meant to happen. Even the things that seem like a 'bad choice' are often, with hindsight, bringing us to the lessons that we need to learn for our awakening and evolution. Life is happening for us, not *to* us. Just because your choices are guided doesn't mean it's all going to work out exactly as you think. Once we get in the mindset of wanting whatever serves our highest good and detaching from the outcome and expectation of this lifetime, we become free.

Do you really have no choice?

While it is common to feel like you don't have a choice in some things, I invite you to start questioning if that is a fact. Do you really have no choice? When I ask my clients this, they often start defending the perspective that they are stuck in their situation, but I encourage them to start seeing that they always have a choice and then acting from that place.

When you feel like a situation is choosing you and you're not choosing it, come back to this concept that you always have choice. When you do this, you attract options. You train your mind to seek solutions, opportunities and creative ways around the situation. In other words, you manifest new choices.

Feeling stuck without choices happens from fearing a backlash or consequence from acting on the choices we do have. Let's look at an example of a relationship that doesn't feel good anymore. We are free humans. If we want to be with someone different or if we want to leave because we are no longer in love with our partner, we have the choice to go. What makes us feel like we don't have a choice? The fact there are massive implications of ending the relationship. If we do something 'out of the norm', such as leaving a partner, there are always consequences. Often, we can't deal with those consequences, because they are too terrifying to contemplate, so we tell ourselves that we have no choice but to stay.

Further to that, if we don't have a healthy understanding of worth, we will also feel that we don't have a choice about staying in this relationship. In the moment, it's not even so much worrying about the consequences, but thinking nobody else will ever love us and that this is the only outcome we will ever get. Childhood trauma is usually playing out here.

Lack of self-worth is usually the driving force behind making choices that don't honour someone. This might look like a reluctance to invest in themselves by going on a retreat, getting to a yoga class, having a healing treatment, investing in coaching. Yet the same people often shop, eat out/order in multiple times per week, go to Starbucks etc, which often adds up to the same sum. The former choices might help a person thrive but it's not always the choice that is made.

Often, we *could* spend our money on what we truly want, but we have competing priorities. We may tell ourselves that we can't afford it, whereas what's really happening is we don't want to deal with the consequences of not having that money to spend on something *else* we feel we need.

Money is an area where it's great to adopt the mindset of choice, remembering that there are always competing priorities, but you aren't obliged to take any of them.

As awareness grows, choice flows...

Week on week, day by day, hour after hour, your awareness grows. It can be confronting when we realise that we have had so much choice all along but couldn't see it. When your consciousness and love expand, you will be able to see that you have more choices because you have learned how to articulate what you need.

When I was a yoga teacher in England, I wanted to go travelling, but I had all these courses booked in. I wanted to do it all! I would think to myself, "Wouldn't it be nice if I could do what I want to do and figure out a way to make it all work perfectly?" With this question in mind, I wrote down on sticky notes everything I wanted to do and stuck them to the wall behind me. Every day, I would look at those sticky notes in a mirror and play this little game where I would try to read them backwards and work out what they said. As I was doing this, I was raising my awareness and using my brain creatively, while staying in the frequency of wonderment and possibility with the intention, "Wouldn't it be nice to figure out a way?"

Then one day, I figured out a way!

I went to India and started teaching online.

There is always a way, but 'the way' doesn't necessarily look like what we think or imagine it will. And it only shows up when we have a level of openness. The magic of life is seeing it all figured out, but the way it comes through is a massive expression of creativity from the Universe. We don't need to know *how*. We just need to know it's *possible*. Because anything is possible, especially when we let go of expectations and trust our intuition. As your consciousness expands, so too will your choices.

PS I Love Me Practice

When talking about higher forces, sometimes it's such a full 'yes' that it's almost like that path is choosing you. In this conscious place, feeling like you 'don't have a choice' is not such a bad thing, because it is a matter of being fully guided rather than trapped by fear of consequences.

How do you know whether you're choosing something out of guidance or fear? Here's an exercise to feel into the difference.

1. Get comfortable and take some deep breaths to settle into yourself.

2. When you're ready, ask yourself this question:

   Why might I be choosing this?

   Think about what benefits you might be getting from staying in this situation and write down what comes up for you.

3. Usually, there is a key lesson that you can extract. Identify what that lesson is now.

   If you can't and you feel like you're completely fixating on getting a specific outcome or maybe that you have 'no choice' in a situation, there may be an unconscious pattern playing out for you. Stay in playful curiosity around this and check in with why it might be happening.

4. Once you find the lesson from a situation in which you feel stuck, your inner world changes. When you

have been completely honest with yourself and can see what's underlying the way you are feeling, ask yourself:

What could I choose instead?

Choices don't have to be completely life-altering to create an important shift. Maybe you just need to tweak some behaviour, the language you're using or set a new boundary.

When we shift our patterns and truly understand what is going on for us, our inner world changes and our outer world follows. That is manifestation.

As a practical example, let's say you're in a job and you work on shifting your inner world to increase your self-worth. As a result, maybe you ask for a pay rise, introduce some boundaries around what time you're going to leave the office, and ensure that overtime is paid at double your rate. When done with self-love, a recalibration takes place. Two paths could open up here. Either your workplace matches your higher vibration and rises to your level. Or it falls away and you find another job. At the time, that may look a little turbulent! However, either consequence is fine because it is coming from a place of self-love. It's all flow.

The same can happen in relationships that aren't going well as a result of a lack of self-love. You can do the inner work, but you must be prepared for the outcome that either your partner is able to up level to match you or they're not. Neither option is easy, but both will ultimately lead to growth. In fact, when I work with single women at the beginning of their self-love journey, I suggest not trying to manifest a partner at the start, because of who they might manifest before they raise their vibe. That's because without raising your vibration, you may attract the same thing over and over until you learn your big lesson. Once they have raised their level of self-worth and learned from some of their past lessons, the partner they manifest is likely to meet them at a higher level.

Bold choices

With love and compassion, sometimes we have to change our circle of influence. This doesn't mean ditching all our friends and family, but it does mean limiting our interactions with people who are not able to support our dreams and visions. This is not easy, but it is rewarding. This is the hero's journey, one where the choices are bold and strong.

To follow your own path, you have to know *why you are doing it*. That clarity of intention will get you out of bed in the morning day after day, ready to move towards your dreams. It is not willpower that will make you take action and push you to make bold choices, it comes from a much deeper place; a profound knowing that this is your purpose and your passion.

When you have a vision and a mission, you don't just choose once. You don't just pick a new path and it all falls into place. You have to keep choosing. Even when times get tough. Even when you are met with obstacles. It is not easy to step out of the box and choose something bold and different. But being clear about your mission will make it easier to push through the stressful, challenging moments that arise.

Often, you won't have anyone to copy or follow when you're on this path. You are a pioneer. You just have to keep on choosing yourself boldly and with self-love.

Good/bad versus *effective*

When we label choices 'good' or 'bad', we approach ourselves from a place of judgment. But when we look at whether a choice can be regarded as *effective*, it allows us to evaluate our choices more objectively. It helps us to remember that we were doing our best at the time and that choices we once considered 'bad' could actually be regarded as *effective* in moving our life forward in a significant way. Moving your language away from judgment towards curiosity, by evaluating how *effective* your choices were, can help to shift your programming into a higher vibrational place.

You are an accumulation of a million choices. You may have felt like other people were making the choices for you, but it's time to remember your power and know that you are the creator of whatever you want, and then some!

Even if your life is not yet transforming as you were hoping it would, stick with it. As you continue to read, little seeds are being planted, even if they are not yet blooming. Everything you need to learn is taking root page by page.

PS Here's Your Self-Love Medicine

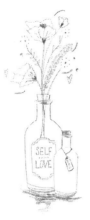

What choices would someone who loves themself make in your situation?

What choices could you make to start loving yourself more?

CHAPTER TEN

Realisation-ships

"Our parents, our children, our spouses, and our friends will continue to press every button we have, until we realise what it is that we don't want to know about ourselves yet. They will point us to our freedom every time."

Byron Katie

Relationships wake us up to our own stories. Given the realisations we can have about ourselves when we're with another person, they should be called realisation-ships! How we relate to others and love others says so much about our relationship with ourselves. This chapter, step ten, is all about that dynamic and how relationships play into the self-love journey.

Lacking love

For the longest time I didn't want a relationship. As a teenager, while my friends were having their first boyfriends and girlfriends, I was into horses and didn't want to start dating. In my late teens,

The truth of our being
just quietly knows and
therefore chooses to not have
to prove anything to anyone.
It resides in the clear, quiet,
grounded place of
understanding self.

PS I Love Me
www.ginaswire.com

I had my first boyfriend, and it was good, but for me, it was never true love. Then in my early twenties, when I was modelling and travelling a lot, I struggled with relationships. I'd have short-term connections wherever I travelled but I always kept men at arm's length. For more than 10 years, I craved romantic love from a man, but I never admitted it out loud and would push love away. How sad is that? I wanted connection and love, but I wasn't available for it, although I didn't know that at the time. As you can see here, I was having an inner conflict and as a result feeling stuck, frustrated and blocked.

It was only when I went on this self-love journey that I realised I had everything I needed inside. This was a surprise at the start! For as long as I could remember, I had thought I would meet a man, some Prince Charming, and he would give me love and I would give him love and we'd be 'in love' and that would be that. I couldn't believe how wrong I had been. No man was going to come riding in on a white horse to save me. I was going to have to save myself. So that's exactly what I did.

I found self-love. Although it was never really about 'finding' it, I *reconnected* with the love that was already there inside me. And I did it by doing everything that I've been sharing over the last nine chapters. So, if you're also craving romantic love, but are still unsure of how to find that self-love within, keep doing these practices and reflections. It's all waiting for you. Just remember the process isn't linear. It's perfectly imperfect.

When it clicked that I needed to love myself first and I started embodying that, less than two weeks later, I experienced love at first sight with an incredible man. Remember how I told you at the beginning of this book about meeting him in India when I stayed to do the advanced yoga training? That's how fast it happened. The two of us were so aligned, and the most beautiful, loving relationship unfolded. I had never experienced a connection so deep. As the love grew between me and this man, I thought there was no greater love possible. It was so big. I did not believe anyone could ever feel more love than this.

As we learn more about ourselves, we become more conscious and our capacity for love expands. This is the concept behind the name of my Facebook group, Infinite Self-Love Society, and my Infinite Self-Love retreats. That expansive love we can feel for someone else all comes from within. As self-love grows, our love for others also matures and grows, getting sweeter, yummier and even more expansive.

Every relationship reflects your relationship with self

Relationships bring up our core wounding, a mirror of everything we have not yet met inside ourselves. Maybe our relationships are distant. Maybe they're dramatic. However they show up, our core wounding is often playing out, yet many of us don't want to look too closely. The themes reflected back to us in relationships can be the same as our own wounds or the exact opposite. Either way, what we see in others can trigger us deeply. This is then compounded by the fact that each party looks at situations with a different perspective and often seeks a different outcome.

Before we go any further, a quick explanation on core wounding. Core wounding is where you didn't get your needs met as a child in some way. This can happen in both loving and traumatic childhoods. When your needs aren't met, it can make you feel somehow *different* to everybody else, although as a human collective we tend to share the same core wounds. Feelings of abandonment, of not being enough, feeling unlovable to a parent, feeling stupid, ugly and unwanted are among the most common wounds, especially in those of us working to love ourselves more.

As described earlier, when my ex and I would have a disagreement, he would want to shout it out (fight mode) whereas I would go quiet (freeze mode). A few moments later, I wanted to talk it all through (appease mode) and he would want to leave and clear his head (flight mode). This was probably so he could calm down and not lose it at me, but it triggered my fear of abandonment. At the time, I thought I was right, and he was wrong. Of course, he thought he was right, and I was wrong. Now I realise that neither of us were right or wrong. We just have different ways of coping and expressing due to our core wounds and how we deal with life!

No matter whether the relationship in question is with your mum, your boyfriend, your friends, or anyone else, every relationship is a reflection of the level of self-love you have reached within yourself. Which is why self-love work is the foundation of creating incredible relationships. And it all starts with the language we use to communicate with ourselves.

When the words you use with yourself come from a place of love, ease, curiosity and joy, you will bring in a loving, peaceful, curious and joyful relationship. Everything that happens with others is a mirror of how you feel about yourself.

Relationships also mirror what is unhealed within us. If somebody is running a story of not being good enough and not being worthy, it is likely their partner is running a story that no partner will ever be good enough for them or show up how they need. Partners' stories often match, like a mirror image, what each person needs to learn. These stories come together to be healed. In the meantime, couples navigate their clashing needs. This might happen through arguments or in conversations where they try to learn from each other. Ultimately, they may come into healing and harmony, but relationships are sent to trigger us.

Take the lessons, wisdom and healing from these relationships, because when you do, you create a beautiful container to fall deeply and truly in love with one another.

As an aside, deep and true love does not necessarily mean a relationship will be everlasting. A relationship can be hugely successful and end at the right time because it does not need to continue for either person. Both of you can thrive after a relationship ends, having gained the beautiful lessons you needed to learn.

Likewise, a relationship does not have to be long-lasting to give you those magical experiences of learning. After my first long-term relationship, I felt like there was a lot I wanted to experience in a short space of time. I manifested five short relationships, not all sexual, not calling them a boyfriend or a partner, because I wanted a learning period with other men who were exactly right for me at the time. These short experiences propelled me forwards in my self-growth.

What does every good relationship need?

If every relationship is a mirror of yourself and you want a good relationship, you will need to make sure that your relationship with yourself is good. Think about how you want your relationship to be with the person you love the most. What does that relationship need in order for it to be a good, effective relationship that you want to be in?

Maybe it needs quality time. Maybe it needs presence. Maybe it needs gifts, thoughtfulness, love, support, date nights. Maybe it needs sex.

What a relationship needs is different for different people and at different times in our lives. However, the bottom line is you need to give yourself what you would want in your relationship with another. The reason you need to give yourself these things first is so that you're not *giving, giving, giving* outwardly, without supporting yourself first. That energy is not a match and becomes draining. Self-care has to come in, because you need for yourself what you need in your relationship.

Take yourself on dates. Give yourself quality time. Be present with yourself. Get good at communicating with yourself. Listen to your needs.

All of these gifts to yourself make for an incredible relationship with you and with others. *You* are a really great place to start if you want to create lasting love.

Losing your sense of self

Hands up if you've ever lost yourself in a relationship? I would guess that 99% of people have experienced this at some stage. Losing ourselves in a relationship is when we have a vision of what we want for ourselves and our life but start to compromise our own needs in order to fit someone else's needs and expectations.

The important point here is to be vigilant when it comes to continuing to follow our vision, our personal quest in life and our passions. Being able to truly honour ourselves while in a relationship, rather than moulding and meshing into what the other person wants, or what they see us to be, takes good self-love and excellent boundaries, but it's oh-so-worth it.

PS I Love Me Practice

Self-love requires us to have strong boundaries, but many of us struggle with boundaries in a relationship. This isn't unusual, so please know we all have work to do.

1. Take a moment to pause here to figure out what your work is.

   Do you have super strong rigid boundaries, and your work is to soften and allow people in?

   Do you have slack boundaries, and your work is to do what it takes not to be a pushover with the person you love?

2. Once you've been really honest with yourself about what your boundaries look like, ask yourself:

   Who in your life would you like to have healthier boundaries with?

Just knowing these two pieces of information is soooo vital as it helps you see what you need more of or less of in order to come into harmony with yourself and others.

Relationships help us to grow. Even if we can walk this path alone and create a life without a partner, if we want to evolve, then realisation-ships are good for that. For some people, this might look like having many relationships, or it might mean being in one solid relationship. Whatever it is for you, any relationship will push you to evolve.

Loving yourself into a relationship

As an advocate of self-love, this is a really important point to mention: you cannot love yourself into a relationship. Self-love must be authentic and genuine, not done *so that you can meet a partner.* When women say, "I need to love myself so I can meet my partner", it sets off an alarm bell for me, because it just doesn't work like that.

We need to love ourselves to love ourselves. We need to feel the love and enjoyment of being alive in our bodies and giving ourselves what we need and nourishing ourselves every day. If we're doing this work so that we can *get* something – in this case, a partner to complete us – it has a completely different energy.

I don't subscribe to the idea of 'the one'. I believe YOU are the one you've been waiting for, and YOU are the one who will be with you 'till death do us part'. That doesn't mean you get one *or* the other, either self-love *or* a partner. Self-love is not a replacement for a partner. Being 'the one' for yourself doesn't mean not going into relationships. It's about knowing that you are the creator of your world and that you have access to the deepest love at all times.

A partner is an incredible *gift* in an already happy life. Two don't become one, but two happy people might come together to enjoy their life together, and that is a match made in heaven.

Some people think that staying single is the answer. In my experience, staying single makes loving yourself easier, because as soon as you enter into a romantic relationship you get to see all your bullshit in the mirror of your partner. How they act is a reflection of you! It can be messy, it can be painful, it can be the full spectrum of emotions. However, hiding away on your own for long periods of time isn't necessarily the best thing for humans. I can remember my mum saying a proverb to me a lot when I was a teenager and I've come to understand just how true it is: "It's better to have loved and lost than to never have loved at all."

Just because you have transformed your own relationship with yourself does not mean the perfect partner will show up. You can be the most fantastic woman doing all the work, showing up for your self-love transformation, really going for it, being so kind, so thoughtful, so empathic, so beautiful, so wise... And you can still manifest a wanker. Just because you manifested a relationship with someone who turns out to be a real challenge or the whole thing is plain rubbish does not mean that is what you are. It's an invitation to look at the pattern that might be on repeat. It could be an invitation to step up to another level by cutting cords with that person and letting them go. It might even be an invitation to stay and work on it, which brings us to the c-word... communication!

Communication and authentic relating

I enjoy communicating and have always thought I'm good at it, but wow, have I gone on a journey with it! As my awareness expands, I have fine-tuned and tweaked the way in which I communicate so that I can speak my truth. Speaking your truth is what communication really comes down to, but before speaking it, we need to know it. As you experience your self-love transformation and feel the truth of these concepts in your body, you may naturally become better at communicating because you know what you want. As self-love crystallises, so does your truth, especially when you know where your boundaries are, relate more to your vision and feel more self-worth and confidence.

Once we know our truth, it's easier – almost inevitable – to speak it. It's a virtuous cycle. When we speak our truth, we feel good, clean and pure. When we don't, we can feel yucky and murky.

The throat is the bridge between the head and the heart. The more we know how worthy we are, the more we are able to voice our needs and feel confident sharing our truth. The more we lean into our sense of self, the easier it feels to express ourselves.

Before we are able to do this, our beliefs might look quite different.

I won't be heard.

Nobody will care what I say.

Nobody will hear me anyway.

I don't know what I'm talking about.

I have nothing important to say.

These kinds of beliefs lessen their grip on us when we are in tune with our truth. They are the stories I used to tell myself, but thankfully I rarely hear these voices now. The odd time I will get a familiar feeling, and become all shy and reserved, but I remember not to judge the one who is shy. She needs love too!

When I talk about truth, I'm not talking about one single truth. Truth is always evolving, like a living, breathing entity. As our awareness expands, we can't look at something through the same eyes we had in the past. What we felt was truth back then might be completely different to what we consider truth to be now.

And so, when you say to someone, "Tell me the truth", their perception might not match your own version of the truth. This is key in relationships, where we not only need to know our own truth but respect the truth of others if we are to relate authentically. To do this, take a moment, take a breath, and drop into your truth. It's powerful and sometimes confronting to listen to where you're at in the moment.

With authentic relating, your focus will be very much on *feeling*. As we have seen, when we go off into story mode, we disconnect from truth. We might recount what we perceived happened and what it reminds us of. However, by staying in the emotion,

If I'm not feeling 100%,
I reassure my body that
she's doing a fabulous job.
That she's kind, healthy,
helpful, loved, trusted,
wanted and free.
I choose how I want
to feel when I enter a room and
usually have a word or phrase to
keep me centred like *"grace"*, *"trust"*
or "worthy with nothing."

PS I Love Me
www.ginaswire.com

we can authentically relate our truth. This can be as simple as, "I feel crap", "I feel confused", "I feel angry" or "I feel happy". This method of authentic relating is a great framework to use with a partner. Getting lost in our stories can create a battle, whereas communicating our emotions gives the other person a chance to understand how we feel.

For example, instead of saying, "You did this, and it ruined my day", which can trigger an argument, you could say, "I was thinking about what happened and I've taken some time to figure out what was going on for me. When this happened yesterday, it made me feel sad and abandoned and a little bit ashamed. I don't know why I'm having these feelings. Maybe it's reminding me of something. I just wanted to let you know that's how I was feeling and it's not exactly how I want to feel. I'd much rather feel…"

When you compare those two ways of relating, you can feel the different energy. There's no right or wrong with how someone feels. All feelings are welcome and human. Allowing ourselves to feel our emotions fully before authentically relaying how we are feeling to a partner, friend or family member can lead to more understanding and connection.

The magic of speaking your truth

When we find our voice and open the throat chakra, we move towards being in our truth and *using our voice.*

For me, this happened when I became a yoga teacher. Before I did my yoga teacher training, I hated speaking in public and would never have spoken on camera. I would rarely speak up, even with friends, and was a bit shy. But when I aligned with my vision by taking the yoga teacher training, I found myself wanting to use my voice.

PS I LOVE Me

There are other ways of working with the throat chakra. Singing and reciting mantras can fire up your throat chakra when you allow a beautiful sound to come out. Screaming, growling and raging can also be oh-so-good. The vibrations these sounds make send messages to the body and help to shift stuck emotions, so using your voice can be highly therapeutic and healing.

It takes practice and you probably won't get to your truth straight away. For me, it took years to authentically relate, because I had a tendency to exaggerate. This came from a fear that I wasn't enough, that I wasn't clever enough or successful enough. When I did some inner work to heal this, I began to catch myself in exaggeration mode and was able to repair it. People respected when I told the truth, even when I had to correct something I had previously said. Repair work can be powerfully transformative.

Equally, it's important to feel into where your boundaries are with sharing. Sometimes someone wants to speak deep truth to you or may ask a personal question where you are invited to share your truth. Please know it is completely up to you whether you decide to do that or not. Maybe you are caught off guard. Maybe you don't have the energy for that kind of conversation. Maybe you're not able to be truthful around that matter just now or it doesn't feel good to you. Sharing your truth is your choice. You can always say that you're not available for this conversation or not available for it right now, but another time.

With certain people, you might find you're more available to be truthful than you are with others. This is completely natural and human. Sometimes, we feel confident and comfortable being ourselves around someone, because they accept us for exactly who we are. Other times, we can find ourselves around people who we feel we need to impress or play down a situation. That's okay too. It may be something to do with one of your own triggers or stories from the past that you have yet to understand. Finding the sweet spot and speaking your truth when you feel comfortable is a practice you will master over time.

As your consciousness expands, voicing all of who you are will become easier and more inevitable.

It's all a growth opportunity

Every relationship is an opportunity to grow. Everything is imperfectly perfect. You are constantly learning. You can make mistakes and take the lessons from them. The most beautiful, painful, joyful, messy experiences we ever have are in relationships. Beauty meets grief meets love meets heartbreak meets joy meets pain meets peace meets misery meets happiness. It's all expansive. It's all evolution. It's all there to serve your soul.

If you are brave enough to love, congratulations! You have experienced impermanence. Nothing lasts forever, but you have been bold enough to go into something with love. Have an open heart and know that all is welcome. All feelings, all communication. Let it all unfold.

PS Here's Your Self-Love Medicine

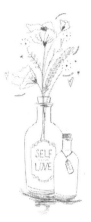

What keeps happening in your realisation-ships?

What would you like to see more of in future or current relationships?

How can you give yourself more of those things now? (hint: #self-love – hehe!)

CHAPTER ELEVEN

Relax! It's Just a Dark Night of the Soul

"The cure for pain is in the pain."

Rumi

Life isn't going to be rosy all of the time and it doesn't have to be. When life isn't going well it can feel like hell at the time, but dark times can turn out to be magical and amazing points of growth.

Having a dark night of the soul is not just for people who have lost their way or don't love themselves. Whether your self-love is strong or not, you can still have a dark night of the soul and go through difficult times. It doesn't look the same for everyone. Some feel depressed, others have a 'crisis' moment, others may not know where to turn. Whatever it is you may be going through, the real question is, how are you going to love yourself through it?

In chapter eleven, we get some perspective on the times you have a dark night of the soul so that you can prepare and have some

As your consciousness expands,
so too will your *choices.*

practical pointers to come back to when you need them. Because dark times are inevitable but having self-love can help you along the growth curve.

Ups and downs

Because humans are cyclical, seasonal beings, we have good times and we have challenging times. Dark periods in our lives can happen for many reasons and can coincide with greater external shifts such as planetary movements, hormonal changes, moon cycles, changes in the collective consciousness and upgrades in your life.

According to Thomas Moore in the foreword to *Dark Night of The Soul: Songs of Yearning for God* by St John of the Cross, translated by Mirabai Starr, we can consider the dark night of the soul like "a crossroads in our effort to make a meaningful life and to achieve a sense of union with the life coursing through us".

A dark night of the soul often happens after an encounter with the divine or when a strong connection breaks. When a rupture happens, we crave the safety of the womb, the security of home. We want to belong again after a rejection, so we seek home. We may experience this like a yearning or a loss, but the truth is we are always home, always safe. We have simply forgotten this which makes us feel as if there is void inside ourselves. But the void is not real. We don't need to fix anything, and we don't lack anything. In time, we will make our way home to ourselves.

Dark periods can feel empty, confusing, even terrifying. You may feel a deep sense of sadness and despair, an acute sense of unworthiness, a longing or yearning, or a mixture of everything. During these times, your will and self-discipline are often weakened, making it difficult to act, and these times are also often accompanied by existential questions.

As challenging as these times may be, they create the opportunity for growth. And as you move through the experience, the principle of contrast means that life can feel utterly wondrous. As St John of the Cross writes, "Souls begin to enter this dark night once God draws them forth from the state of the beginners, who merely muse about the spiritual path, and places them in a state of the adepts, the true contemplatives. This is the start of a journey that will lead to the blessed place of perfection, which is the divine union of the soul with God."

A dark night of the soul is fertile ground for our deepest awakenings, where we meet ourselves in our deepest despair. The all-encompassing darkness is an invitation to enter the abyss, for us to jump into everything we've avoided or are most scared of. It's where we take huge leaps forward in our spiritual growth and remember the love within ourselves. It's a powerful spiritual platform from which to evolve.

Zooming in, zooming out

As we've established, dark times feel incredibly difficult when we are in them, but I would like to offer a little perspective here. As little humans living our little lives, it often feels like everything revolves around us, but when we zoom out and look at what is happening on a cosmic level, we can see our stresses and strains for what they really are. While they can feel overwhelming as a little human, it's helpful to remember that we are a teeny speck on a tiny planet in an infinite cosmos.

To do this, when you're feeling overwhelmed or stressed, try going outside and looking at the sky. If it is daytime, look up at the clouds and see how expansive it all is. If it's night, look up at the stars and see how powerful they are. This is not to bypass our troubles, but simply to gain a touch of perspective.

When we zoom back in, we might realise that our human selves are actually a bit safer, healthier and more secure than we feel. If we have a home, some money, some friendships and are somewhat supported, even though things might feel like they're not working, there are usually ways in which we are also very lucky and blessed. When we become fixated on what we lack, it's important to take note of the basics and connect to gratitude for what we do have, because we are so lucky to even just be safe.

Impermanence

Another way of looking at dark times is to focus on the impermanence of it all.

Our troubles or challenges can perpetuate if we let them. Imagine a day where you wake up and feel a bit flatter than usual. Maybe you didn't sleep well or maybe you had some weird dreams or maybe you don't have a clue why you feel down. When we start to analyse why we're feeling how we're feeling, it's a form of attachment to the feeling of difficulty and it perpetuates. Likewise, we may start off with an unhelpful thought about our body not being good enough and that thought quickly becomes contagious. Suddenly our relationship isn't good enough, and our work isn't good enough, and so on... Or maybe we'll binge on crap food which makes ourselves feel worse and then it perpetuates that way. Down, down, down the rabbit hole we go.

Sometimes these things are happening for a reason and are exacerbated by the environment. I've already mentioned that planets and hormones and collective shifts can play into that escalation. Sometimes, though, these things are perpetuating because we have latched onto them and that attachment creates the struggle.

Remembering the cuteness hack can be a huge help when we are attaching to the struggle, because cuteness can't coexist with criticism. When your cute little human is struggling, it's time to look at yourself in the mirror and remind yourself that you're really doing well. Acknowledge that it's a hard time for your cute little human and praise her and thank her for persevering through the crappy, rotten time.

It's important to mention how tricky this can be to do in the moment. It doesn't feel cute at the time – when you're in it, when everything sucks, when you're lying on the sofa, when you're crying, when you want your mum, or your dad, or your partner who is no longer in your life, when you can't see the light at the end of the tunnel – you can't always feel the 'cute'. You probably can't feel anything hopeful. You just want to know if this dark time will ever end.

Please know, it will end. Everything is impermanent. Everything passes eventually.

"This too shall pass" is the most underrated of all the inspirational quotes out there!

During the times when everything that you normally practise isn't working and you can't seem to feel better and love yourself, remembering the reality of impermanence can be very reassuring. It will pass. It will not last forever. You will connect again.

Turn your trauma into dharma

One of the most inspiring ways I have been taught to conceptualise dark times comes from a friend, Silvia Mordini, who believes that the people who experience the darkest times are the ones who expand most into their light and go out into this world to teach and share the message revealed to them. If we want to learn, to transform, to teach, we must embrace our darkest parts and 'change our trauma into dharma'. When I heard this phrase, it resonated deeply with me, because I realised that every teacher I know who is involved in transformational work has been through incredibly challenging times in their lives.

So, what is dharma? There are many ways to describe it and I remember there being a debate around exactly what it is when I was doing my training in India. In my interpretation, which I take from the way I was taught, dharma is where you are living your life purpose or mission in harmony with highest good for all. And of course, self-love can lead you to this calling or mission. This is the definition we'll use for the purposes of this book.

Healed trauma can help us find the message that we want to share with the world. It's worth saying here that some people say it can take a lifetime to heal trauma. I have not found that to be the case in my own experience or that of my friends and clients. If we believe that we have a lifetime of 'work' to do, then we will expand that work into a whole lifetime. Just like that idea that if we have a week to pack for a holiday, it takes us a week, but if we book a last-minute holiday and have 30 minutes to throw a bunch of things into a bag, we get it done pronto (speaking from experience here!). The task expands to fit the space you give it.

A friend of mine, Abi, was having severe digestive problems that were to do with emotional trauma and a lack of self-love. One day, she said to me, "It has taken 30 years to get into this mess. It'll take me a long time to get out." I questioned this. Was that a fact? Did it have to take all that time? When she thought about it, she realised she was telling herself a story, and thus, not healing. As soon as she realised that it didn't have to take a lifetime, she not only healed her digestion, but also started an amazing new business and rekindled her connection with her amazing husband.

That's not to say trauma will dissolve overnight. Getting good quality advice and support is essential. I have had a lot of help reaching this point myself and it's what I now offer clients.

To even begin to heal your trauma and turn it into your dharma, you'll need to understand it. Trauma is any event that 'exceeds our capacity to cope emotionally'. That could be something as simple as being told we are fat by another child or losing a parent in a supermarket and feeling abandoned.

In the example of the child losing their parent in the supermarket, even if they weren't really alone or abandoned because the parent was just in the next aisle, a child may not have known that. As children, we internalise traumas and they can live on. The child who believed they were left in the supermarket might have thought they were never going to see their parent again, that it was their fault and that they were unlovable. Trauma is anything that meets us in a place in our lives where we don't have the tools to cope. It isn't just what happened to us, it's how what happened affected us and changed our way of relating to the world. Of course, the point here is not to compare our traumas to anyone else's, but to point out that challenging events can be transformed into our teachings.

For me, this was being with my dad when he died. This was a trauma and an honour and a turning point in my life.

It was a trauma because I was 'losing' a primary caregiver, a super special person in my life, and watching him pass from the world I live in. I will never ever see him again in this human form. That's the unknown, scary and painful part.

It was an honour because I got to experience the whole 'mind-body-soul' thing. One minute his soul was in his body; the next, his body was an empty shell. I got to witness his transition. That was something I'd never wanted to see, but when I did, it was actually

Self-love

is not a replacement for a
partner. Being "the one" for
yourself doesn't mean
not going into relationships.
It's about knowing that you are
the creator of your world and
that you have access to the
deepest love at all times.

a beautiful and powerful moment for me. It was an honour to be present for him too. He knew his family were all around him and I hope he knew how much we all love him. I'm in tears as I write this, yet I smile because I know he would be so happy to be mentioned in this book. He was such an inspiration to me and a massive part of this self-love movement, which helps so many, even though he's all the way out there in heaven! Thank you.

When he died, I remember feeling relief, joy, peace and stillness. It wasn't at all like I would have predicted. I went to the window of his house, which overlooked his garden. I could see every blade of grass in high definition. It was like I'd put on 5D glasses. I could see the edges of the clouds and different colours I'd never seen before.

Seeing my dad die at 54 was a catalyst for change in my life. It woke me up and I am forever grateful for that. I no longer wait to do the things I love. I no longer plan things far away in the future. I live life to its fullest now. Work hard so I can retire and have fun? Nope. Go and have fun now. Fun helps manifest magical opportunities. Freedom helps manifest incredible opportunities. Happiness and fulfilment create miraculous opportunities. Life is happening now. It's definitely no dress rehearsal.

Friends and family, especially my mum, moved me through the loss of my dad. The night that he died, I said to my mum, "I don't know what to do with myself."

"What do you want to do?" she asked.

"I want to go out and dance," I replied.

"Well then do that," she said.

So, I did.

I remember it so clearly. We danced salsa all night in a bar in my hometown of Poulton-le-Fylde. And it really helped.

The message here is powerful. What do you *want* to do? Give yourself permission to do that. You know what's best for you. I'm lucky and grateful to have such a beautiful family who love me unconditionally and are happy when I'm happy. Deep down, I believe their souls know that I'm on this special mission and they know I need to be free.

Around the time of my dad's passing, I made a number of realisations around my purpose, and my path, and what I was born for. It showed me that I have a limited time on this earth and have to make the most of it because nobody is going to do it for me. When he told me not to wait and that life is not a dress rehearsal, I took it very literally. Now, I don't wait. I rarely say, "I'll get to that next time." I make it happen straight away!

Not only did my dad's passing ignite this urgency in me, but it also made me more compassionate, as a person and as a coach. It put me on a path to health and healing that led me to do the work I'm doing now. Experiencing dark and challenging times was essential to becoming a self-love coach, because I realised how everybody goes through their own stuff. It taught me to feel deeply for everyone, to understand what people are going through and to have respect for where people are on their journey with their pain.

I also felt my spiritual connection strengthening, and for that I'm massively grateful. I wish for everybody to feel that level of cosmic support for themselves.

We can be grateful for dark times because they bring incredible messages, lessons and wisdom that we may pass on. We teach our scars.

Even if it feels counterintuitive to be thankful for dark times going on in your life, hang in there. You don't need to do anything. It will pass, but the more you resist, the longer it might persist. Feel it all, because one day, you will know why you went through what you're going through now, and you'll be able to take it forward in your life and mission. You're in the dark so you can understand the light. This is the path of initiation.

Laughter is medicine

I want to end this chapter by giving you an important tool for dealing with the darkness, and that is to approach it with laughter and light. When everything feels like it's caving in and crumbling, you can feel disconnected and terrified. We have all asked ourselves at some point, "Is this ever going to end?"

If you can, try to encourage yourself to have a bit of a laugh at how crazy this time is or take some time to physically shake it off. Doing this will up your vibration and be good for the nervous system. It will raise your frequency, which will help you move through it.

Even in the mess, do not abandon yourself. Never stop being there for yourself, being your own best cheerleader, loving yourself.

You might be at rock bottom, begging for a sign on the kitchen floor, but always, always have your back. Be there for yourself. Remind yourself that you'll always be there and that you are amazing. Believe what you're experiencing is making you a kinder, more compassionate, more caring, more expansive person; this will help get you through.

The longer you stay in resistance and try to push away dark feelings, the harder it will become. Likewise, trying to carry on as normal, shoving it away, eating, drinking and shopping to numb, numb, numb, will lead to energy getting stuck in your body. If you can allow the dark feelings to be there, have a good laugh, have a good shake, have a good dance, move the body, move the emotions, have gratitude for this dark time, then the light will return. Without darkness, we wouldn't be able to appreciate the light.

PS I Love Me Practice

Using a mix of what I've suggested above or other support that you feel will help you, make a survival plan for how to get through dark times.

What can you do today that will soothe or help you?

What can you do this week?

Do you need more support right now? If so, who do you know or what do you need to research to help you on that deeper level?

For instant calm, you can also check out my *What to Do When You Lose Your Shit – Guided Visualisation* at www.ginaswire.com/bookresources.

CHAPTER TWELVE

Passionfruit

"Your greatest self has been waiting your whole life; don't make it wait any longer."

Steve Maraboli

When you've cleared a lot of the BS about yourself, revisited and upgraded the unhelpful thought patterns and beliefs, you can go after what you want in your life! Fully guided by self-love. You also tend to get introduced to your divine mission. It happened to me, and it happens to my clients and friends when they embrace the concepts I've shared with you over the course of this book.

That juicy passion-fuelled life is available to you right now. You may already feel it. If you're still thinking that it can't happen for you, *trust* me on this one! It *will* happen for you too. And the best part is that living this way is the most powerful and self-loving thing you can do!

Living a passion-fuelled life, fully in your power, means you're manifesting, you're making money, you're in the flow, you're

Feel it all, because one day,
you will know why you went
through what you're going
through now, and you'll be able
to take it forward in your
life and mission.
You're in the dark so you can
understand the light.
This is the path of initiation.

creative, you're happy, and you're surrounded by good people and experiences. You're on top of things, you're dedicated, you're owning it all. It sounds like a dream and a place we would all like to be, so how do we learn to live in this place?

In this final chapter, we answer that question and explore what it really means to step into your power and live a passion-fuelled existence.

The problem with power

Often, I am asked: *How can I be in my power every single day?* It's a question that has baffled me in the past, firstly because we are always in our power and secondly because there are always going to be times when we don't feel very powerful, and that's okay. We can all feel disempowered, so trying to feel powerful all the time is impractical.

What I think people mean when they ask me that question is: *How can I show up for myself every single day and stay aligned with my highest good?* These 12 steps to a self-love transformation are filled with tools to help you create and maintain a loving state. What it always comes back to is reconnecting to your highest self or inner knowing.

The other aspect I think people are getting at when they ask about power is: *How do I move from a disempowered state into an empowered state?* The problem with seeing power as something you can lose or gain, is that you forget that your power is always within you. If you're feeling disempowered, it's about first looking at ways to reconnect to your innate power.

Before we look at how to reconnect, let's look at what's going on under the surface, and why we don't step into our power every single day.

Power blockers

There are a few reasons why we may not step up to claim our power and knowing what they are can empower us beyond measure.

Unprocessed trauma

Unprocessed or unaddressed trauma is probably the most important piece here because it creates a lack of clarity, focus, awareness, and generates fear. When pieces of ourselves are completely detached from our power, usually this has happened as the fallout from an event that gave us the first experience of feeling unworthy or disempowered.

When we look at the history of our own lives in detail, we can understand why we feel the way we do. Once we have this awareness, we can heal and thrive.

Fear of success

Self-sabotage happens to us all. We reach a certain point and then we give up. Imagine you were trying to get healthy. For a while, life would be all about going to the gym, eating the fruit and veg, drinking water, avoiding the sugar and foods that don't work for you. Maybe you start to feel good, but then suddenly you find yourself deciding to do something unhealthy. Maybe you go get drunk and eat pizza and a kebab on the way home.

Why do we do this? Why do we see it all going so well, then 'fall off the wagon'? It's partly because we fear our own greatness. If we are so great, so fantastic, so successful, so beautiful, so healthy, so rich, our ego can get nervous of it all being taken away. Our ego likes to keep us small and safe, so that we are not abandoned.

If you suddenly make a huge leap, where does that leave partners, friends or family? This is hugely scary to our little human selves. It's not fear of failure. It's fear of the unknown. It's fear of success, the greatest fear humans know.

Clarity

Another reason why we don't step into our power is a lack of focus or vision. If we are trying to do something but do not know why, we can flounder. Having a vision or focus that is crystal clear gives us direction and a path to follow.

Making constant decisions without knowing our direction takes a lot of energy that we could be using to step into our power. Instead, we're directionless and lost. Even though we may feel like we know what we're doing, if clarity is an issue, if our direction is not a firm, clear YES, we can get stuck.

Imposter syndrome

God created everyone equally. Nobody is more worthy, more important or more capable of love. However, some of us become disconnected from our gifts, often because of the way in which we are conditioned to not stand out. As children, we are taught (directly and subtly) to stay in the box. Shame might come into play here. Have you ever been or seen a child who is larger than life being put in their place? Told not to sing or dance? Told not to dress creatively or express their emotions deeply? Children who are charismatic or 'out there' may be taught to fit in, told to 'wear the uniform' and conform. This conditioning disconnects us from our uniqueness and willingness to stand out and shine.

When we are trying to step into our power, it is common to question ourselves and our legitimacy. Known as imposter syndrome, this can be devastating to our confidence and can keep us small. It often occurs when we compare ourselves to others and ask, "Who am I to do this when there are so many amazing people doing it better than I could?" In other words, "Who am I to be so confident and to shine?"

Who are you to do this? Well, who are you not to do it? You are no less than anyone, than Richard Branson, than Oprah Winfrey, than Beyoncé, or whoever is killing it in your industry. We can all take up the same amount of space in the world.

Feeling like we don't know what we are doing and staying in that comparison space prevents us from stepping into our power, but this is a choice. In reality, everything is available to us.

Awareness

The last main reason that we don't step into our power is a lack of awareness. If we don't know who we are, if we don't understand our emotions, if we don't know how to ask for what we want, if we don't know how to create a vision, if we don't know how to use that vision as guidance, this lack of awareness makes stepping into our power much more difficult.

One aspect of awareness is the very concept that we always have power. Some people struggle with that notion, but it is vital to embrace in order to connect with the power within.

If you are struggling to believe that you always have power, here's an image that might help. Imagine the sky. We know that the sun is always shining, but sometimes we just can't see it because of where we are standing. If we are on the ground and there are clouds in the sky, they block the sunlight from reaching us. We know that the sun is still there, but the clouds are in front of it. The sun doesn't go away, but we can't always 'connect' with it. Self-love doesn't go away. Power doesn't go away. Self-love and power are always there. It's just about removing the clouds.

Healing is messy

Stepping into our own power means seeing *all* parts of us, including the dark corners within us. It means accepting and healing the parts that are fragmented and misaligned. Being brave and diving into these aspects of ourselves attracts healing, opportunities and evolution. The willingness to be real, bold and honest with ourselves is how we rise.

When you first step into your power, it doesn't mean everything will go well all at once. Having it all together is a myth. Indeed, becoming empowered can look really hard at first.

Stepping into your power is way more subtle than you might be imagining. Even though I was empowering myself by stepping away from a career that no longer resonated with me, when I first left modelling, I actually felt lost, directionless and passionless. While I no longer had to try to be someone I wasn't, when I stepped into my power and walked away from it all, I was lonely, desperate and terrified. I would be on my lounge floor in tears, begging for a sign, feeling like shit. That is *not* the picture of empowerment we imagine! What we think of when we talk about 'stepping into our power' is a state of manifesting, having amazing opportunities, being in a state of receiving, love and open-heartedness, and taking up space. But what it really involves is reclaiming the parts of yourself that you may have rejected.

On the outside, it may even look like disempowerment, because healing is messy, but this is a necessary step if you are to move into flow, create from your passion and attract amazing opportunities. Manifesting incredible things may be a side-effect of stepping into your power, but empowerment is much more than that.

Power is when we stop being a victim. It's when we stop wondering why everything happens *to* us and realise it's happening *for* us. It's when we start having boundaries, self-worth and self-love. It's

PS I LOVE Me

being playfully curious about your belief systems and reflecting on the places you are staying small or feeling a lack of choice.

What disempowerment looks like

Disempowerment looks different for everyone and can be hard to recognise when you're in a rut. However, bringing some awareness and energy to these areas is going to reconnect you with your own love. If you recognise yourself in any of the behaviours listed below, please try not to judge yourself. We all have days that look like this, so just know that this happens to us all. When I have days like this, I love to 'take a zero'. This is where you clear your diary and order in everything you can possibly need to have the comfiest day of your life doing sweet nada. This can be one of the greatest self-love gifts you can give yourself. But it only works if you let yourself *receive the rest* without feeling guilty. Giving yourself space to rest and integrate can be one of the most *productive* things you can do. Whereas feeling guilty for looking after yourself gives your power away, and the loop continues.

When we're not in our power, this can look like:

- Not doing your usual practices, even though you know they will help you

- Not wanting to do that project you were excited about, but don't feel good enough to do

- Finding evidence that this low-vibe state is true

- Moping around, spending or wasting time in a brooding, listless state due to being upset, unhappy, dejected

- Being low-vibe (linked to fear, anxiety, sadness and depression)

- Overly relying on other people to soothe us instead of self-soothing

- Attaching to stories that you tell yourself are negative

- Half-assing it in relationships

- Finding issues everywhere you look

- Wearing pyjamas all day (when it doesn't feel good, not because you've consciously chosen to have a lovely slow self-care day)

- Not showering until dinnertime, because you want to wallow in your own despair.

Stepping away from disempowerment...

When we feel this way, there is plenty we can do to reconnect with our power. Here are a few solid ideas of practices to get you started.

Coming back home

Coming back home to yourself can be as simple as breathing or meditating. Close your eyes right now and breathe down into your tummy. Let your jaw and stomach relax. Do about 10 deeeeeeep breaths in through your nose and out through your mouth. It's sooo super simple but brings you home every time. Don't skip it! Your body will thank you.

Creating space

Overwhelm, struggle and disempowerment are just a perception, but it can be hard to see a way out until we get some space. Take space for yourself to start seeing more clearly. Book a 'Me Date' in your diary right now. Put an hour or more aside just for you where you have unstructured time to look after yourself. Make

Giving yourself space to

rest and integrate

can be one of the most
productive things you can do.

PS I Love Me
www.ginaswire.com

a commitment with yourself to give yourself this gift (I do this regularly). In this time do something nourishing for yourself, turn off your phone, go for a walk, journal, be still. Whatever you feel like doing. This only works if you do it!

Physical and metaphysical clearing

Take some time to clear out your physical and energetic space; this could include your wardrobes and your belief systems. Address your circle of influence and check in to see if there are people or physical items that no longer work for you.

Refocusing

Stop focusing on everything that is out of alignment with the life that you want to have and instead give your energy to what you *do* want. Write a list of what is working and what's not working for you. Be gentle with yourself.

Remembering

Remember the truth: everything is perception, and you always have a choice about how you feel inside and how you relate to any situation – how empowering is that to know?! Let that land within you!

... towards empowerment

Now that you have created some space from your feelings of disempowerment, we are going to look at how to reconnect to the power that is always within. When we are fully in our power, we are in a state of manifesting, making money, bringing in amazing opportunities and feeling in a flow state.

You can make the choice to step into your power on a daily basis. Every day, you have the choice. Think about it. It's a knock-on effect. You wake up, make the choice to feel empowered and

BOOM, you head to your wardrobe and pick up a sexy little number, you head out feeling like a sassy little minx, you stand a little taller, your heart's a little more open; the pavement feels like a catwalk, you're fierce and ready to slay. All from that one little empowerment tweak you started your day with.

I believe every human is born with a mission. We all have something to bring to this planet, our Goddess-given gifts, and it is our life's work to share them. We are here to be in service to the world. If we are not showing up, not finding our gifts, not sharing our wisdom, not revelling in our uniqueness, we don't get to share our contribution, which is a shame for us and a shame for the world.

Sharing our gifts is true empowerment and every single one of us can do that. We all have experiences and gifts that we can share. Sharing your Goddess-given gifts, practising those gifts, teaching from your experience, sharing from what you know, that is where your power resides. FYI – it's crucial to share your own authentic gifts rather than copy someone else.

For that, you need to go within and connect with your mission, quieten the mind and listen to your heart.

Ring, ring! It's your *calling* calling

Throughout *PS I Love Me*, I have talked about having a vision and mission for your life. Mine is to help a billion women to feel self-love and get everything they want in their lives. Yet for years, I didn't live with passion and I had no idea what my purpose was. For 30 years, I didn't even know I had a calling.

Some of my passions are adventuring to random places all over the planet, experiencing different cultures and rituals, being part of healing ceremonies, holistic health, crystals and witchy magic! I also love nothing more than holding dinner parties for friends, going to the market and spending hours choosing food and cooking it, then feeding people and sharing wisdom around the table. Nurturing is something I do in my business too, but before my passions and purpose found me, I spent my fair share of time partying and floundering around, wondering what I really was going to do when I grew up.

If, like me, you are a slow developer in this domain, or don't yet know what your passion or calling is, you can listen in, look back, connect the dots and create space for your intuition to guide you, AKA letting go of the good to receive the great. I truly believe that your calling chooses you. When it finds you, you will know about it! And the Universe will conspire in your favour. And it's important to note that you're not limited to just one mission. Like in my favourite movie *Interstellar*, you might have a main mission and lots of sub-missions. Just like relationships are often described as 'for a reason, a season or a lifetime', missions can be the same. We are constantly evolving and so are our missions. And remember to have fun with it all!

Spend time doing what lights you up, what feels fun and joyful, what feels effortless. When you do that, you'll meet people who light you up because they love to do that too. And you'll find yourself in the right places at the right times. This is how the Universe conspires in your favour. Follow the breadcrumbs!

Breadcrumbs are always there but we aren't always willing to see them. Maybe you're just sitting there thinking, *"Why are there all these breadcrumbs?"*

Here's an example of following the breadcrumbs and the Universe conspiring in your favour to help your calling find you.

Imagine you love whitewater rafting, so you go on holiday to a place where you can do that. That's a breadcrumb. You do some rafting, and you love it. You think, "This would probably never be my career, but it really lights me up." While you're there, you meet people who teach rafting, and they tell you how they made it a career by opening a rafting place. That's a breadcrumb. Maybe they ask you to help out while you're there and you offer to volunteer during your holiday. Breadcrumb. Turns out you're quite good and the owner offers to pay you for your time. Breadcrumb. The company needs someone to take pictures at this certain spot, which sounds fun to you, so you take them up on it. Breadcrumb. You really enjoy it, so you decide to take a course in outdoor adventure photography. Breadcrumb.

Before you know it, you become an international freelance extreme-rafting extraordinaire! All because you followed your passion. Honestly, it can be that simple.

If you're still unsure, let me recap my own journey of following the breadcrumbs to create the purpose-led life I have today.

In the beginning, I was a bit unhealthy and wanted to learn about nutrition, so, as I mentioned at the start, I enrolled in a course but quickly discovered that it wasn't at all what I was aiming to study. The Universe had a different plan. But the course was *fun*, so I stuck with it. Breadcrumb. During the course I decided to open a coaching practice, all about food, which I *love*. Breadcrumb. To complement this business, I taught some healthy cookery lessons and found I really enjoyed the experience of *teaching*. I thought of opening a cookery school, but it didn't feel quite right which led me to consider what did feel right. Breadcrumb.

I was passionate about yoga, so I went to India and took a yoga teacher training course. That felt *really good,* and I learned loads and met amazing people. Breadcrumb. Some of those people who I met in India lived in Bali, and that led me to visiting Ubud which *instantly felt like home.* Breadcrumb. Becoming a yoga teacher was rewarding but I had a strong sense that it was *just a fraction* of what I had to offer to the world. Breadcrumb. And then it hit me, self-love had *TRANSFORMED* me. It felt like the Universe really wanted me to build this self-love community. I wasn't planning it, it planned me! Breadcrumb, breadcrumb, all the breadcrumbs! Actually, the full loaf!

A few years ago, I learned the term 'multipotentialite' which resonated with me deeply (check out the awesome TED talk by Emilie Wapnick). From childhood we're constantly asked what we want to be when we grow up, which can create a sense of panic and pressure. People who don't know what they want to do and don't have a clear answer to that question often begin to feel 'less than'. I used to feel that way. But then I realised that, by darting around the world following my desires, I've picked up so many amazing skills which are now fundamental for my work as a self-love mentor.

Now I hold self-love retreats, organise online events, speak around the world and am interviewed on TV and in magazines, I can now see how my degree in event management, my experiences on camera and travelling the world as a model, my love of nourishing people by serving epic food and my crazy yogic adventures in India have all come together to serve my mission for the good of all womankind. All because I followed the breadcrumbs and made some serious dough on the way, hehe!

That's passion and that's purpose. It doesn't even have to be your career at first, if that takes the pressure off. It never needs to be forced. It only needs to be followed. Forcing yourself along a path can take you way off-piste, which I see with friends who went into corporate jobs just because they paid well. They are now stuck paying for a whole host of expensive habits, designed to distract them from the lack of joy and fulfilment in their working lives. No amount of Sky Plus, designer dresses or passionfruit martinis will make up for a job that lacks true passion and purpose. It's all about choice. And knowing you have that choice in every moment is what empowers you.

There will be fear and risk and judgment from others when you follow your passions to find your purpose. There may even be a fair amount of investment. You will have to make choices and may be faced with unsupportive people, but that is totally okay. It's okay to take risks and not quite know why, so long as it is guided by your passion. Maybe the worst thing that can happen is you have to come home and get a job because something didn't work out. Many people are scared they will fail, but if failure looks like coming home and getting a job, which is where they are in the first place, it makes perfect sense to try, at least, doesn't it? At this point in humanity, we need everybody who is willing to get out of their own way and step up so that we can ascend to a higher consciousness.

Circle of inspiration

I recommend surrounding yourself with inspiration and listening to the wisdom of people you aspire to be like. Get a coach, a circle of influence and role models who are already doing what you'd love to do. At the same time, limit how much you pay attention to the views of people who you don't aspire to be like.

To be the hero of your own story and live a completely free life, I suggest listening to the advice that resonates with your passion and calling, the people who you see to be constantly free in themselves and their lives, the ones who are not afraid to share with you that their lives aren't perfect all of the time, who are conscious, who are in service to the world.

If you don't have a passion and purpose yet, it's about exploring more and listening in to yourself. That means exploring deep within your heart and also exploring this beautiful planet we live on.

Exploration and adventure have been some of my most powerful teachers. The university of life. The university of Pachamama in all her gloriousness.

I want you to know that you do have that choice, you can make huge transformations and you have the power within you to pursue anything you want to do. It's totally possible. I see it day in, day out. We are infinite beings living in an infinite Universe. Because limits are imposed by self, they can be removed by self. It starts with you. You are the creator of your reality and the faster you realise how powerful you are, the more enlightened and peaceful this planet becomes for us all. Imagine yourself rockin' it in your rocking chair as a glorious wise woman, having broken the patterns of self-criticism, disempowerment and restriction once and for all. Passing on this new paradigm of light language to the next generations and watching the world become the place we once wished for.

PS Here's Your Self-Love Medicine

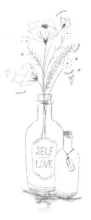

Here's to living a powerful, passion-fuelled, purpose-filled life!

Visualise the most empowered version of you, sometime in the future when you have overcome your challenges. How does she think, walk, talk to herself in the mirror, make choices?

Now that you have read this book, what are three things you have realised about self- love?

What is your vision for the year ahead?

If you're ready and raring to get going, check out *How to Create a Badass Vision Board & Start Manifesting Your Dreams* at www.ginaswire.com/bookresources.

PS... AN INVITATION
TO GO DEEPER

"Fall in love with where you are.
Turn towards this – a sacred moment,
unrepeatable. Trust the ebb and flow of
things. Say yes to uncertainty and the
unresolvedness of your life. Come out
of stories and second-hand dreams and
remember the place where breathing
happens. Here. Now."

Jeff Foster

You've made it through the 12 steps to self-love. You've come all this way. You've read the wisdom, owned the stories and done the work.

And now, here's one last little piece from my heart to yours. If you've reached the end, but you've half-assed some of it or skipped the bits you didn't want to face, go back in and give yourself this gift. Cutting corners on your self-love journey doesn't serve anyone and nobody else can do this for you, so dive back into the chapters and make sure every box is ticked, every concept grasped.

You are the creator
of your reality
and the faster you
realise how powerful
you are, the more
enlightened and peaceful
this planet becomes
for us all.

PS I Love Me
www.ginaswire.com

I said at the beginning that you can do this your way. And I really meant it. There's no 'right way' to have a self-love transformation. The journey doesn't end here. The self-love journey will last a lifetime. Whenever you feel the need, you can keep coming back to the book and finding another lesson depending on where you're at in your life. There's always more to unravel, more to learn and more to be gained. As your life unfolds, different lessons will speak to you more powerfully, and that's perfect. There's so much juice in these pages, but as humans, we can only take one sip at a time.

Whenever I go back to something that I've learned before, I realise how quickly we forget the transformations we've previously had. So, remember to look back at how far you've come. You'll always get a 'repeat' transformation as you remember the lessons you learned back then and realise how they apply now that you've reached a whole new level.

You are where you are

The other important thing to leave you with is the sense of letting go of the need to 'do the work'. Learn the concepts and then let them go. Don't attach to them. Don't take them too literally. See what feels right for you. Use the bits that work. Take whatever you wish, apply what resonates and leave the rest. This will be different for everyone.

Also know that confusion is inevitable! There is a duality in this work. Everything is right and wrong, so part of the process is accepting this duality and using what is true for you in any moment. This slight confusion is actually a great place to be because it allows you to make up your own mind, which is what we're working towards anyway.

Always remember, when you think you've 'cracked it', there's more. There's always more. In a good way! And when you think you've lost your shit, that's often when these enlightening feelings come in, so go with it.

It's all happening for you... and you get to choose!

If that's hard to grasp on a human level, think of it on a soul level. Your soul is choosing this for you. The ideas in this book are already integrating within you, even if you don't feel it, see it or sense it yet, know that it is done.

We are all on the journey back home, back to ourselves, back to alignment. Back to our natural state, which is and always was, of course... self-love.

NEXT STEPS

Loved the book and would like some accountability? Craving connection with like-minded women? Wish you could work through these steps live with me? Your wish is my command!

Introducing the 12 Step Self-Love Transformation course!

If you are craving more interaction, my 12 Step Self-Love Transformation course is curated especially for you, so you can continue to deepen your transformation with me and create a life beyond your wildest dreams. The course includes epic video trainings covering the 12 steps in easy manageable chunks, worksheets and checklists, bonus resources, downloadable MP3s, a private Facebook group support centre and four live coaching calls with me. It's the gift that keeps on giving!

You can expect to experience:

- More confidence

- Deeper, more soulful relationships

- More opportunities and wealth

- More vital energy than you knew was possible

- Enjoying being in your body more than ever!

- Find out more at www.ginaswire.com/my-12-steps

Retreats and Coaching

Alternatively, if you want the VIP treatment so you can squeeze loads more extra juice out of your self-love journey, why not join me on one of my transformational retreats and get an in-person experience? Retreats and events run in the UK and Bali, so keep up to date with what's happening at www.ginaswire.com/events or over on Instagram www.instagram.com/ginaswire/ where I love to share the latest on all things self-love!

ABOUT THE AUTHOR

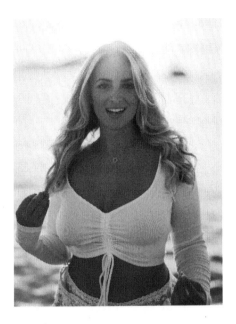

Gina Swire is a self-love mentor and manifesting queen on a global mission to help a billion women fall madly in love with themselves. After struggling with her own self-worth and image issues, Gina quit her career as a plus-size model at the height of her fame in order to embark on her own journey of transformation.

Today, she travels the world leading live workshops, hosting retreats, coaching private clients, speaking on international talk shows and stages from Burning Man to Bali. Gina's work has been featured in *Vogue, Cosmopolitan, Elephant Journal, Yoga Guide Magazine, Psychologies*, Burning Man and Bali Spirit Festival.

Since 2014, Gina has been teaching self-love in a variety of formats from one-to-one coaching to group programmes, retreats and live events. She has coached thousands of women on self-love. And now she's written the book on it!

Gina's coaching draws on a wide range of modalities and life experiences. She is a certified health coach and a life coach, as well as 500hr advanced registered yoga teacher and meditation teacher. Having immersed herself in this topic, she teaches her signature 12 steps to self-love and how to do the deeper work.

Gina inspires women everywhere to love themselves and love their lives. Learn more about Gina and become a part of this self-love movement at www.ginaswire.com.

Space to write your self-love notes

Space to write your self-love notes